CARING FOR A LOVED ONE

WITH ALZHEIMER'S OR OTHER DEMENTIA

— PAPERBACK EDITION —

EVERYTHING I WISH I HAD KNOWN

LEAH STANLEY

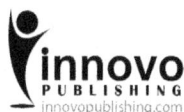

innovo
PUBLISHING
innovopublishing.com

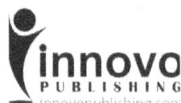

Published by Innovo Publishing, LLC
www.innovopublishing.com
1-888-546-2111

innovo
PUBLISHING
innovopublishing.com

Publishing quality books, eBooks, audiobooks, music, screenplays & courses for the Christian & wholesome markets since 2008.

Caring for a Loved One with Alzheimer's or Other Dementia
Everything I Wish I Had Known

ISBN: 978-1-61314-915-7

Cover Design & Interior Layout: Innovo Publishing, LLC

Printed in the United States of America
U.S. Printing History
First Edition: 2023

Has God called you to create a Christ-centered or wholesome book, eBook, audiobook, music album, screenplay, or online course? Visit Innovo's educational center (cpportal.com) to learn how to accomplish your calling with excellence.

CONTENTS

The contents of this book have been incorporated into two online courses:

1. **The Professional Continuing Education (CE) Caregiver Course** is certified for social workers, nurses, and certified case managers. The course covers the day-to-day needs and available resources for primary caregivers of loved ones with Alzheimer's or other dementia. To learn more and take this course, scan the QR code or place the following link into your browser: https://bit.ly/ce-course

2. **The Individual & Healthcare Organization Caregiver Course** is designed for individuals caring for a loved one and for healthcare staffers who want to be prepared to support their organization's clients who are primary caregivers (but don't need the continuing education credit). The course can be accessed by individuals, or group registration can be arranged. To learn more and take this course, scan the QR code or place the link below into your browser: https://bit.ly/caregiver-course

WELCOME!

Welcome to *Caring for a Loved One with Alzheimer's or Other Dementia: Everything I Wish I Had Known.*

It's been a minute since my book *Goodnight, Sweet: A Caregiver's Long Goodbye* was first published. That's good because now I've had time to sit back and take a deep, cleansing breath. Writing the book meant I had to step back into my "caregiver" shoes and walk again through the flood of emotions piqued by the experience of being an advocate for my grandparents. Now I am able to engage in reflection, and I regard with amazement how God brought me through the rigors of caring for two people who had been severely short-changed by Alzheimer's and unspecified dementia, respectively.

When my caregiving journey began in January 1997, I had *no* idea what I was getting into. All I knew was my wonderful grandparents, for whom I had so much love and affection, desperately needed my help. In my heart I was glad to do anything I could for them, but back then the things I *didn't* know about elder care could have filled the Colosseum in Rome; my ignorance of the subject was just short of debilitating.

I didn't know the difference between Medicare and Medicaid. Had I been asked to differentiate between independent living, assisted living, and a nursing home, I might have come up with only broad definitions and vague guesses as to what they were and how much each one might cost. And when it came to my grandparents' money, I had no idea who, if anyone at all, I might ultimately have to answer to regarding how it was spent. Additionally, the phrase "durable power of attorney" held no meaning for me whatsoever.

From an emotional perspective, I was completely unprepared to process the reality of my grandparents' dementia symptoms. Time after time I would throw all my energy into doing anything I could for them; and time after time, doing so would drain my mental reserves until finally I would hit a wall and melt down in tears. I didn't know whether my feelings and experiences were normal or weird, and because I was the designated caregiver it was always *my* signature on every document, and I perpetually carried the weight of everything that signature set in motion.

I discovered one particularly unpleasant part of the job was having to deal with distant family members who didn't really want to get into the messy business of actual caregiving, but they were very eager to register their complaints and/or get in line for a potential inheritance.

And then there was having to tell and re-tell the story of how I came to be my grandparents' legal caregiver while I was still only twenty-nine years old. I understood it was a part of the caregiver's role to answer the questions of various relatives and health care providers alike, but the odd looks and furrowed brows which came as I explained that my grandparents' own son had abandoned them always made me feel embarrassed and ashamed; the discussion became irritatingly redundant because it never got easier.

Occasionally, though, I would run across someone who had experienced something similar to what I was going through; being able to talk with people who knew *exactly* where I was imparted a refreshing breath of air into the monotonous isolation of caregiving. There was something eminently comforting about connecting with those who had travelled that road before me, and I would grab on to their words as we compared notes on shared experiences, clinging to them as if they were life preservers thrown to a drowning soul.

Goodnight, Sweet: A Caregiver's Long Goodbye detailed my passage through the world of elder care where I was dogged by doubt and uncertainty, even as I was crying out to God for Him to lead me and make the way clear. I give all glory to His great Name because the way *was* made clear, but only one step at a time. It is my sincere hope that the book will show people there is a way through the wilderness of caring for an afflicted loved one, and that my readers' fears, doubts, and insecurities will grow pale and fade away as confidence is placed in Jesus, relying on His Spirit to chart the path forward; as Jesus said in John 16:13a, *"But when He, the Spirit of truth comes, He will guide you into all the truth...."*

Now, drawing information from my own caregiving background, I have developed *Caring for a Loved One with Alzheimer's or Other Dementia* to allow light into the maze of pain and uncertainty faced by those who provide care for others. I had a breadth of experience to draw from, including navigation of medical and federal insurance benefits; discovering why the power of attorney needed to be a "durable" one; learning that all Alzheimer's is a form of dementia, but *not* all dementia is Alzheimer's; and comprehending that "therapeutic lying" is not a form of deception but rather a peaceful means of survival for the patient's family.

Through the pages of this book, I'm going to walk with you as I would a close friend, talking about things I wish I had known when I started to care for my grandparents. I'm not a lawyer or a counselor or a medical professional. I am an experienced Alzheimer's/dementia caregiver—I've walked this thing out. So let's you and me engage in an open, honest conversation about this great blessing, this dreadful mantle: the tidy mess of caregiving.

CHAPTER 1

LET'S TALK LAW

I n this chapter we will,
- Examine why establishing an estate plan matters
- Define legal document options for an estate plan
- See that funeral preplanning is part of a good estate plan
- Consider the benefits of having a will or a trust

Benjamin Franklin said, "If you fail to plan, you are planning to fail." As we delve into the world of elder care, one of the first issues to be tackled is just that: establishing a plan that will protect you and your family as everyone continues to age.

There are a variety of reasons people don't plan ahead for their estate or personal care needs: some people get busy, assuming they have lots of time left and they'll get around to it later; others are superstitious, thinking if they start drafting documents to provide for themselves in the event of the unthinkable, then the unthinkable event might actually occur; then there are those who simply don't know what to do, and so, feeling completely overwhelmed, they do nothing.

Whatever the reasons may be, a good way to push past them is for you to understand what can happen if there is no plan in place at all.

THE ABSENT PLAN

> *"You know," Dr. Weston began, "you're lucky. You've come in here with all the right papers in legal order. Because of that you'll be able to take proper care of [your grandmother]. You're lucky she thought ahead and did this. Let me tell you, we have people come in here all the time just like your grandmother and we can't do a thing for them because they haven't appointed anyone to make decisions for them."*
>
> **Excerpt from *Goodnight, Sweet: A Caregiver's Long Goodbye***
> **Chapter 8: "Admission"**

If a person suddenly (or in the case of one of the dementias, *not* so suddenly) becomes incapacitated and they have not pre-appointed someone to make health care and/or financial decisions for them, a family member can petition the court for **guardianship**—also known as **conservatorship**.

That person will then need to have the ward (the one needing the care) declared **incompetent** as determined by a qualified physician.

> In law, the term incompetent refers to a person's inability to understand legal proceedings or transactions or lack of mental capacity to understand the consequences of his actions.[1]

Difficulties may arise if there is more than one family member who wants to have input regarding care for the ward, or who wants a say in how the ward's money is being spent. If no one seeks guardianship, the court itself may appoint a family member to serve in that capacity. In certain situations, such as having no family member available, physicians at a medical facility can make decisions pertaining to the health care of the ward, but it may not be in line with what the ward might wish.

Something else to consider is that once the courts get involved, all records and proceedings are open to the public. This means the family's personal, private, and sometimes painful matters can wind up on display for anyone to see. On top of that, any court costs and legal fees can be taken away from the assets of the ward's estate, meaning that at the end of it all there may be very little, if any, inheritance left for the ward's heirs.

Regardless of how it comes about, a court-appointed guardianship can be a time-consuming and costly process; just getting started with court filing fees, hiring attorneys to represent both the ward and the one seeking guardianship, as well as paying for any medical reports required by the court can run into thousands of dollars very quickly. There can also be ongoing fees and costs after the guardian is appointed.

One final thought pertains to the ward's available cash in a checking or savings account: having no pre-appointed agent can mean that management of the ward's finances may wind up being turned over to the state in which the ward lives.

Whether you're taking care of yourself or someone you love, the bottom line is this: in order for anyone to ensure that both their financial and health care needs are handled in accordance with their wishes, *every individual* needs to take the proper precautions well ahead of time; don't wait for a crisis to hit and then find yourself (or your loved ones) scrambling for the right thing to do.

---

1. www.legaldictionary.net

THE LEGAL DOCUMENT BUFFET

"Well," Bruce paused pensively. "Fortunately for them and for you they took the appropriate legal precautions. They have each prepared a legal document which gives durable power of attorney to a specific person pre-appointed by them….Both of them appointed you as their only alternate agent….The term 'durable'…indicates these papers are not affected by the incapacitation of your grandparents."

Excerpt from *Goodnight, Sweet: A Caregiver's Long Goodbye*
Chapter 5: "Legalities"

When I first met with my grandparents' lawyer, Bruce Hollis, he released to me their original durable **power of attorney** (POA) documents which had been prepared almost five years earlier. I learned the term **durable** was very important; it meant the authority they granted me to act on their behalf was *not* affected or compromised in any way by their respective dementia diagnoses.

> Power of attorney (POA) refers to the granting of authority to one individual to make decisions for, and to act on behalf of, another individual.[2]

For the sake of clarification, let's look specifically at my grandmother's documents. Grandma (known in her legal documents as the *principal*) had prepared a durable POA, which is a type of **advance directive**. In it, she appointed Grandpa as her agent to make decisions for her in the event of her becoming incapacitated. If for any reason Grandpa was not able to serve as her agent, she had appointed me as her alternate agent; it turned out to be a very good thing she had me designated as a back-up because Grandpa wasn't able to serve for her since he, too, was incapacitated by an unspecified form of dementia.

> An advance directive is a legal document in which the signer (also known as the principal) gives directions or designates another person to make decisions regarding the signer's health care if the signer becomes incapable of making such decisions.[3]

In their individual durable POA documents, both of my grandparents outlined and ensured my authority to take proper care of them in every situation; that one document covered everything from the disposition of

---

2. www.legaldictionary.net
3. www.thefreedictionary.com/advance+directive

their property and finances to their health care and end-of-life choices, including the "**Do Not Resuscitate**" (DNR) order.

A second form of advance directive used in estate planning is the **living will**. Whereas the durable POA grants authority to an assigned individual who will make decisions for and act on behalf of the principal, the living will is a document that allows the principal to specify what their wishes are with regard to certain life-sustaining or life-saving procedures; basically it outlines what you do or do not want done, but *it provides no authority* for anyone to act as your agent on your behalf. Both are advance directives (as shown in the graphic below), but they differ in their scope and limitations.

Advance Directive

Durable Power of Attorney	*Living Will*
(Names a person who has authority to act for you)	(Merely states what you do or don't want done)

There are other more specific types of power of attorney documents, including a **nondurable POA** (usually drafted for a specific legal or financial goal). The nondurable POA will automatically end if the person who made it becomes mentally incapacitated. There is also a POA for health care and a separate POA for finances. A parent may decide to give a POA for health care to one adult son or daughter and give the POA for finances to another. Splitting up the responsibility may be a good idea, depending on the strengths and weaknesses of the people involved.

My grandparents' estate planning documents, drafted and used more than twenty years ago, were very competently put together; they each had a single document which gave me authority over anything that had to do with them. However, as times have changed, so has the way these documents are drafted. Today, a complete estate planning package includes individual documents to address specific areas:

- Statutory durable power of attorney
    - ¤ Covers personal business issues, but nothing medical
- The living will
    - ¤ For physicians and family; it will indicate your desire regarding the DNR order and whether or not you want to be connected to any type of life support

- Medical power of attorney
  - ¤ This authorizes your agent to make health care decisions for you if you are incapacitated
- The HIPAA (Health Insurance Portability and Accountability Act) release form
  - ¤ To ensure your designated agent has access to your medical information from your physician
- Last will and testament
  - ¤ To be enacted upon your death, designating how your estate is to be disbursed between your heirs

These documents may vary from state to state, so it is best to speak with an attorney to make sure you understand what specific forms you may need. Often an initial consultation with an attorney is free of charge, so I encourage you to take advantage of that opportunity to learn more about how you can effectively protect yourself and your family.

THE FINAL DISPOSITION

On the day they were admitted to Waverly, Audrey had reminded me I could spend down their money by updating their funeral arrangements....I did [find] an envelope with information about arrangements at a funeral home in Memphis....I was encouraged to upgrade their caskets....[I] learned they had not pre-paid for a police escort, nor had they purchased the floral display...which would lie over the lids of their caskets.

Excerpt from *Goodnight, Sweet: A Caregiver's Long Goodbye*
Chapter 17: "Financial Responsibilities"

To augment the estate plan for you or a loved one you are caring for, I urge you to consider including pre-arranged funeral instructions. Regarding my grandparents, I discovered they had already made the bulk of their own arrangements. They had paid for services at a funeral home in Memphis, and they had purchased two side by side graves at a cemetery owned by the same funeral home. They had even ordered a dual headstone in advance.

Once my grandparents were admitted to Waverly Nursing Home, I had to spend down all their available cash to an acceptable limit so they could receive Medicaid (something we'll cover in greater detail in chapter three). Because I understood the average cost of a funeral could easily run into thousands of dollars, I knew it would be best for me to finalize these arrangements while they still had enough money to pay for it.

A funeral or memorial service involves many choices, including which funeral home to use, making the decision between burial or cremation, the selection of a casket or an urn, and whether to have a minister or a simple eulogy by a family member. If a burial is selected, you may need to invest in a police escort if the grave site is not located near the funeral home where the service is held. When you add in the selection of flowers, music, and potential speakers, you have the makings of an overwhelming task. Whatever your preferences may be, the most important thing is for you to communicate your wishes, or, if you are providing care for someone else, make sure you're clear on how they want to be memorialized. It will be far less stressful to discuss these elements ahead of time rather than waiting until you or your family members are weighed down by grief.

To Will or to Trust?

With Grandma's passing, I knew that I had also been released from my legal role as her appointed agent with durable power of attorney. It was now time for me to serve my grandparents one last time as the executrix of Grandma's last will and testament.

Excerpt from *Goodnight, Sweet: A Caregiver's Long Goodbye*
Chapter 24: "Release"

One of the most important documents a person can ever put their signature on is their **last will and testament**. Many people think having a will is only necessary if there is a large estate or a vast sum of money involved. The fact is, no matter how much "stuff" you have, it's *your* stuff, and you have the right to say who gets it after you're gone.

If you were to die **intestate**, meaning without a will, your estate (defined as all your tangible possessions, your real property, and the cash you have in any bank account in your name) would be put through a **probate** process, and it would be distributed to beneficiaries based on the law set forth by the state in which you owned your property. Most wills do go through probate, but it tends to be more expensive to go through an intestate probate process than it would be if you had prepared a will, and usually the court costs are taken out of the value of whatever property the heirs would inherit.[4] In short, your heirs lose out if you don't prepare a will.

---

4. "What Happens When There is No Will or a Lost Will?" laws.com, modified December 22, 2019, probate.laws.com/will/what-happens-when-there-is-no-will-or-a-lost-will

Probate is the legal process of transferring a person's property to beneficiaries or heirs after death.[5]

The only criteria for making a will is that you must be of legal age (eighteen in most states) and of sound mind. In the document, you must specifically name the people or organizations you want to be the recipients of your money, property, and/or possessions. In addition, you will need to name an executor (also called an executrix), someone whose job it will be to see that your wishes are carried out.[6] The term **executrix** is somewhat antiquated; simply put, it refers to a woman who holds the executor position. It still appears in legal documents from time to time, but the term **executor** is more commonly used to refer to either a male or a female in the role.[7]

One important thing for you to understand about the probate process is that it can be brutal on a deceased individual's bank account—with *or* without a will. In order to protect funds that are in a bank account, it is best if the owner of the account fills out a "**payable on death**" (POD) form.[8] It works like this: as long as the account owner is living, the individual they've named to inherit the money in the POD account has no right to it at all, but upon the death of the account owner, the bank will release any and all funds in the account to the pre-named beneficiary, and it will completely bypass probate court.

Another estate planning option for you to consider is the establishment of a **living trust**. A trust allows you (known as the **settlor**) to appoint another person or an organization such as a bank (known as the **trustee**) to oversee property and/or finances for the benefit of a third party (known as the **beneficiary**). It is referred to as "living" because it's created now, while you are alive.[9] It can go into effect as soon as it's created, unlike a will which can only go into effect after your death.

There are a number of reasons a living trust (rather than—or in addition to—a will) may be chosen to supplement a family's estate planning needs. A trust has the ability to protect minor children by appointing a trustee

---

5. www.legaldictionary.net

6. "Requirements for Making a Will," UpCounsel, UpCounsel Technologies, Inc., 2022, upcounsel.com/lectl-requirements-for-making-a-will

7. Julie Garber, "What Is an Executor?" The Balance, Dotdash Publishing, updated October 25, 2021, thebalance.com/executor-executrix-3505523

8. Mary Randolph, J.D., "Payable-on-Death (POD) Accounts: The Basics," Nolo, MH Sub I, LLC, dba Nolo, accessed February 2022, nolo.com/legal-encyclopedia/free-books/avoid-probate-book/chapter1-1.html

9. Christine Fletcher, "9 Reasons Why You Should Consider a Living Trust," Forbes, August 16, 2018, forbes.com/sites/christinefletcher/2018/08/16/9-reasons-why-you-should-consider-a-living-trust/?sh=6531aec835df

who can not only provide care and guardianship for the child(ren) but can also make decisions for the benefit and protection of the minor(s). Having a trust can also allow the heirs to avoid probate, which, as we discussed earlier, can be a lengthy and potentially expensive process; additionally, a trust can better protect family privacy because wills usually become part of the public record whereas a trust is a private document.

One thing people have asked me is whether or not they should have a lawyer draw up their estate planning documents. It is true that a host of legal documents are available on the internet, and if they are notarized, they can get the job done; my maternal grandmother's documents were done that way. My mother had no problems because there were no other living heirs, so when her mother died everything that remained of her estate came to my mother without question.

However, I must confess that I was very glad Grandma and Grandpa had had their documents drafted by a bona fide attorney. There were multiple heirs to my grandparents' estate, but because I knew their lawyer had drafted documents that had been tailor-made for them, I had the confidence to act on their behalf without fear, never wondering if their documents would be able to stand up to any scrutiny.

One final thing to consider is once you have your documents prepared, be sure to store them in a safe place. My grandparents kept all their original documents in their lawyer's office, and they provided me with copies for my own records. It would be wise for you to keep copies of all your documents in a wall or floor safe or in a fire-resistant lock box, and you might want to make sure you provide copies to anyone you've designated to act on your behalf.

In conclusion, let me state emphatically that *I am not a lawyer*, and it is not my intention to give you legal advice. My goal is to get you thinking about your estate planning needs and to give you a brief overview of some options you have. Whether you are looking at providing care for aging parents or if you realize that you yourself don't have anyone appointed to take care of your business and make decisions for you, I urge you to establish a proper estate plan immediately. It is also important to periodically review your plan to be sure it remains "up to date" and able to adequately meet your elder care needs because life circumstances are subject to change.

If you would like to see an attorney but aren't sure where to find one, start by checking with your church, or talk to a trusted friend who may be able to refer you to their attorney. You *can* establish a solid estate plan, and its benefits will one day be a blessing for both you and your heirs.

QUESTIONS FOR CONSIDERATION

1. Who would you rather have make decisions for you: someone you appointed because you trust them, or someone appointed by the court—someone who may not see *you* as their first priority?

2. You've spent your lifetime working to build your "nest egg." Would you rather see that money and/or property go to your children, your grandchildren, or some other person of your choosing, or would you want your inheritance for them eaten up by probate court costs and attorney fees?

CHAPTER 2

MEDICAL MATTERS

I n this chapter we will,
- Define "dementia"
- Identify the four most commonly diagnosed dementia types
- Examine "sundowning"
- Review the tests used to establish a dementia diagnosis

Having to provide care for someone who is afflicted with any type of sickness awakens a demand for answers to questions like, *What is happening to my loved one?* and, *What can I do to help them?* Whether the illness is manifesting as mental or physical, the need to identify the condition, establish a treatment plan, and understand the eventual prognosis weighs heavily on the mind of the caregiver. Expectations will inevitably develop from information provided by members of the medical community, and it will be supplemented by people we know who have had similar experiences.

Most medical professionals would agree that an accurate diagnosis is the first step in getting a patient the help they need. Because my grandparents' issues were primarily mental in nature, this chapter will focus on diagnosing and treating patients with symptoms related to a variety of dementia types. It is noteworthy, however, that the protocol of identifying a problem then establishing a course of treatment seems to be the universal path for all forms of illness, both mental and physical.

IT WAS 1995, BUT MARILYN MONROE HAD JUST DIED?

Clearly something was wrong, but I hadn't known what to do about it. Each time I talked with [Grandma] she seemed to be a little worse than the time before, and I would come away feeling utterly helpless.

Excerpt from *Goodnight, Sweet: A Caregiver's Long Goodbye*
Chapter 1: "The Message"

While visiting Grandma and Grandpa during the summer before Chris and I were married, Grandma asked us if we had heard about "the actress who had died." We asked her who she was talking about, and we could see she was struggling to come up with a name.

"She was blonde," she said, "and she committed suicide. I don't remember what else they said."

We looked at each other puzzled. We knew of no one fitting that description who had been in the news regarding a suicide or even an accidental death. Then Chris gave me a knowing look and asked Grandma, "Are you talking about Marilyn Monroe?"

"Yes," she said. "That was the name."

As people age, it's not uncommon for memory to be affected to one degree or another, but hearing Grandma talk that day about Marilyn Monroe's death like it had just happened—even though thirty-three years had passed since the actual event—left me wondering what was going on with her. When circumstances finally necessitated that she and my grandfather be examined by a physician, I learned they were both suffering from different types of **dementia**—a general term for the loss of memory and other mental abilities caused by physical changes in the brain; these losses are significant and severe enough to interfere with daily life.[10]

In our society people frequently joke about their forgetfulness, laughing as they say their Alzheimer's is acting up. The truth is, Alzheimer's is only one of several different types of dementia, and its diagnosis is *no* laughing matter. It is *not* part of the normal aging process; it's vastly different from the garden variety "forgetfulness" that all people experience from time to time. Researchers have identified many[11] different types of dementia, including these four which are the most frequently diagnosed:

1. **Alzheimer's Disease:** A degenerative brain disease, the cause of which is still unclear;[12] it results in problems with memory, thinking, and behavior; it accounts for roughly sixty to eighty percent of all dementia diagnoses.[13]

2. **Vascular Dementia:** A decline in thinking skills caused by conditions that block or reduce blood flow to the brain (such as

10. "What Is Dementia?" Alzheimer's Association, accessed February 2022, alz.org/alzheimers-dementia/what-is-dementia

11. "Types of Dementia," Dementia Understand Together, Health Service Executive, accessed February 2022, understandtogether.ie/about-dementia/what-is-dementia/types-of-dementia/

12. "Alzheimer's Disease," Merriam-Webster, Merriam-Webster, Incorporated, accessed February 2022, merriam-webster.com/dictionary/Alzheimer's%20disease

13. Paula Ford-Martin, "Types of Dementia," WebMD, WebMD LLC, Medically reviewed by Jennifer Casarella, MD, on September 29, 2020, webmd.com/alzheimers/guide/alzheimers-dementia#1

a stroke) which deprive brain cells of vital oxygen and nutrients; this is the type that was referred to as "hardening of the arteries" by past generations.[14]

3. **Lewy Body Dementia:** A type of progressive dementia that leads to a decline in thinking, reasoning, and independent functioning because of abnormal microscopic deposits that damage brain cells over time; it is considered the third most common cause of dementia.[15]

4. **Frontotemporal Disorders:** Caused by progressive nerve cell loss in the brain's frontal lobe (behind the forehead) or its temporal lobes (behind the ears).[16]

Alzheimer's Disease

In 1906 a German physician named Alois Alzheimer presented a case history of a fifty-one-year-old woman who suffered from a rare brain disorder. A brain autopsy identified the plaques and tangles that are now recognized as being characteristic of Alzheimer's Disease.[17] For many years an autopsy was the only way to definitively diagnose Alzheimer's, but today a physician can diagnose Alzheimer's with ninety percent accuracy while the patient is still living.[18] Issues start mild and get worse over time.

- *Symptoms*: Confusion about location or what day or year it is, problems speaking or writing, losing things and not being able to find them, showing poor judgement, as well as mood and personality changes.[19]

14. "Health," Johns Hopkins Medicine, The Johns Hopkins University, The Johns Hopkins Hospital, and Johns Hopkins Health System, accessed February 2022, hopkinsmedicine.org/health/conditions-and-diseases/dementia/vascular-dementia#:~:text=Vascular%20dementia%20is%20a%20disorder,vessels%20that%20supply%20the%20brain

15. "Lewy Body Dementia," Alzheimer's Association, accessed February 2022, alz.org/alzheimers-dementia/what-is-dementia/types-of-dementia/lewy-body-dementia

16. "Types of Dementia," Alzheimer's Association, accessed February 2022, alz.org/alzheimers-dementia/what-is-dementia/types-of-dementia

17. Esther Heerema, MSW, "How Alzheimer's Disease Was Discovered," VeryWell Health, Dotdash Publishing, updated June 21, 2020, verywellhealth.com/who-was-alois-alzheimer-how-was-alzheimers-disease-discovered-3858664

18. Alissa Sauer, "How Alzheimer's is Diagnosed," Alzheimers.net, A Place for Mom, Updated August 13, 2019: alzheimers.net/how-is-alzheimers-diagnosed

19. Paula Ford-Martin, "Types of Dementia," WebMD, WebMD LLC, Medically reviewed by Jennifer Casarella, MD, September 29, 2020, webmd.com/alzheimers/guide/alzheimers-dementia#1

- *Treatment options:* Medical professionals are able to help patients maintain mental function and manage behavioral symptoms through the use of several prescription medications approved by the U.S. Food and Drug Administration,[20] but currently there is no cure for Alzheimer's.

Vascular Dementia

Also referred to as **Vascular Cognitive Impairment**, this dementia type can be brought on by inadequate blood flow, resulting from a major stroke or a series of mini-strokes. It is widely considered the second most common cause of dementia after Alzheimer's, accounting for about ten percent of all dementia diagnoses.[21]

- *Symptoms* include confusion, disorientation, trouble speaking or understanding speech, and vision loss.[22] Symptoms may be most obvious very shortly after a major stroke and can vary widely depending on how severely the blood vessels are damaged and the area of the brain that is affected.
- *Treatment options:* At present, there are no available treatments that can repair the damage once it's happened, but the diagnosis provides the opportunity to prevent further damage.[23]

Lewy Body Dementia (LBD)

Discovered by Dr. Frederic Lewy, this dementia type is an "umbrella" covering two specific diagnoses: (1) Dementia with Lewy Bodies and (2) Parkinson's Disease Dementia. LBD is associated with abnormal deposits of a protein called alpha-synuclein in the brain. Diagnosing LBD can be difficult because indicators can appear similar to brain disorders like Alzheimer's or psychiatric disorders like schizophrenia.[24]

- *Symptoms:* These protein deposits, referred to as "Lewy bodies," affect chemicals in the brain which cause changes leading to

20. "How Is Alzheimer's Disease Treated?" National Institute on Aging, U.S. Department of Health & Human Services, accessed February 2022, nia.nih.gov/health/how-alzheimers-disease-treated

21. "Vascular Dementia," Alzheimer's Association, accessed February 2022, alz.org/alzheimers-dementia/what-is-dementia/types-of-dementia/vascular-dementia

22. Alzheimer's Association, "Vascular Dementia."

23. Joanne Barker, "Vascular Dementia," WebMD, WebMD LLC, Medically reviewed by James Beckerman, MD, FACC, June 14, 2021, webmd.com/stroke/guide/vascular-dementia#2

24. "What Is Lewy Body Dementia? Causes, Symptoms, and Treatments," National Institute on Aging, U.S. Department of Health & Human Services, accessed February 2022, nia.nih.gov/health/what-lewy-body-dementia-causes-symptoms-and-treatments

problems with thinking, movement, behavior, and mood.[25] The patient with LBD might also experience hallucinations.[26]

- *Treatment options:* There is no cure, but some symptoms may respond to treatment for a period of time. Antidepressants can be used to treat depression or anxiety, both of which are common in LBD.[27]

Frontotemporal Disorders (FTD)

Also an "umbrella" term for a diverse group of disorders, FTD affects areas of the brain generally associated with personality, behavior, and language; portions of the frontal and temporal lobes of the brain "atrophy" (shrink), and usually the cause is unknown.[28]

- *Symptoms* may vary greatly from one individual to the next and can include inappropriate actions, lack of judgement, repetitive compulsive behavior, aphasia (the loss of a previously held ability to speak or understand spoken or written language), and movement disorders such as tremor, poor coordination, or difficulty swallowing.[29]
- *Treatment options:* At present, there is no cure for FTD, but symptoms may be managed through the use of antidepressant and antipsychotic medications. Patients experiencing language difficulties may also benefit from speech therapy.[30]

AGITATION AS THE SUN GOES DOWN

I gathered the hangers from the closet and began to put her clothes back.... Then her gaze locked on what I was doing. She came over to me, seized hold of the dress in my hand, and snatched it away from me with one quick jerk.

"I told you, I can't stay here!" she blurted out aggressively.

"Why not?" I demanded....

25. National Institute on Aging, "What Is Lewy Body Dementia?"

26. Susan Bernstein, "What Is Lewy Body Dementia?" WebMD, WebMD LLC, Medically reviewed by Christopher Melinosky, MD, June 7, 2021, webmd.com/alzheimers/guide/dementia-lewy-bodies#1

27. National Institute on Aging, "What Is Lewy Body Dementia?"

28. "Frontotemporal Dementia," Mayo Clinic, Mayo Foundation for Medical Education and Research (MFMER), accessed February 2022, mayoclinic.org/diseases-conditions/frontotemporal-dementia/symptoms-causes/syc-20354737

29. Mayo Clinic, "Frontotemporal Dementia."

30. Mayo Clinic, "Frontotemporal Dementia."

"Because this is Mr. Fred's room!...I'm a lady...and I can't stay in Mr. Fred's room!"

Excerpt from *Goodnight, Sweet: A Caregiver's Long Goodbye*
Chapter 15: "The New Normal"

You may have noticed as the afternoon progresses and the evening is coming on, your loved one with dementia may begin to exhibit a new and more intense agitation as their mood shifts from pleasant and workable to anxious and demanding. They may seem even more confused than usual, and the darker it gets, the more irritable, disoriented, and suspicious they become. They may yell or pace and may even have hallucinations, and getting them to calm down may seem like an impossible task. What's actually going on here?

This late-day mood shift is known as **Sundowning**.[31] Its cause is unknown, but it affects up to one in five people who have Alzheimer's, and there are a number of factors that seem able to trigger it. If the patient is over-tired, or if there is low light and there are increased shadows in the patient's room, Sundowning may begin to occur; or it may be caused by a disruption of the body's "internal clock,"[32] which is the part of the brain that signals when a person is awake or asleep. This area breaks down in the Alzheimer's patient and is therefore viewed as a possible explanation for Sundowning.

The activities and attitudes associated with Sundowning can be very disconcerting for the caregiver. Behaviors such as mild agitation can potentially be worked around, but what about the patient who strikes the assisted living director in the face with his fist? Or the one who breaks the window to "escape" their safe care environment and winds up flagging down a driver on the busy road in front of the building? Sundowning can produce disturbing and potentially dangerous behaviors, so what can a caregiver do to reduce the effects of it?

- Keep things calm in the evening
  - ¤ Close blinds or curtains
  - ¤ Turn on lights around the room

- Try to keep background noise to a minimal level

---

31. Brenda Goodman, MA, "How to Manage 'Sundowning'," WebMD, WebMD LLC, Medically reviewed by Christopher Melinosky, MD, December 29, 2021, webmd.com/alzheimers/guide/manage-sundowning

32. Jonathan Graff-Radford, MD, "Sundowning: Late-Day Confusion," Mayo Clinic, Mayo Foundation for Medical Education and Research (MFMER), mayoclinic.org/diseases-conditions/alzheimers-disease/expert-answers/sundowning/faq-20058511

- ¤ Turn the TV down
- ¤ Seek to reduce the stimulating activities of other family members moving around

- Give the dementia patient a big lunch and then keep their evening meal smaller and simple
  - ¤ Give sweets and caffeine only in the morning
  - ¤ Offer healthier alternatives later in the day

It is important for you as a caregiver to control your reaction if your loved one is Sundowning. You need to keep as calm as you can and ask if there is anything you can do for them. *Do not* argue with them, and if they need to pace or walk around the room, let them do it as long as they are safe. Your continued reassurance that everything is OK might also help. Be sure you discuss this issue with your loved one's physician because they may be able to make recommendations based on their professional knowledge of the patient.

IDENTIFYING THE ENEMY

"[Dr. Carlton] gave [your grandmother] what we call a 'twenty-point quiz' this morning. It's very basic information: Who is the president? What year is this? What is your address?—that sort of thing....Your grandmother scored a seven."

Excerpt from *Goodnight, Sweet: A Caregiver's Long Goodbye*
Chapter 9: "Seven and Nine"

If you are concerned that your loved one may be suffering with some form of dementia, it is best to have them examined by either their primary care physician, a neurologist (a doctor trained in brain conditions), or a geriatrician (a doctor trained to treat older adults).[33] When checking for any type of dementia, medical professionals will combine evaluations that include the patient's history, a physical exam along with laboratory tests, and neuropsychological testing. Despite all the research to date, there is still no single test used to make a dementia diagnosis.

Assessment for any dementia type can include extensive evaluation of memory and thinking skills, lab tests (including blood work, often to rule out other disorders with symptoms similar to dementia), and imaging techniques, such as the following:

33. Mayo Clinic Staff Writer, "Diagnosing Alzheimer's: How Alzheimer's Is Diagnosed," Mayo Clinic, Mayo Foundation for Medical Education and Research (MFMER), accessed February 2022, mayoclinic.org/diseases-conditions/alzheimers-disease/in-depth/alzheimers/art-20048075

- **MRI** (Magnetic Resonance Imaging) which creates a detailed view of the brain
- **CT scan** (Computerized Tomography) which provides cross-sectional images of the brain
- **PET scan** (Positron Emission Tomography) which uses a special dye containing radioactive tracers; it can allow doctors to distinguish between different types of degenerative brain diseases.[34]

Dementia can affect any of the core mental functions:

- Memory
- Language skills
- Ability to focus and pay attention
- Ability to reason and problem solve
- Visual perception[35]

A formal diagnosis of dementia requires that at least two of these areas be impaired.

Being told that a loved one has any form of dementia is devastating; but being able to look the situation in the eye and call it by its right name can be a big help as you seek to understand what your new role as a caregiver looks like. Research is ongoing, but for now, society waits for a cure, and in the interim it's the caregivers who are on the front lines.

QUESTIONS FOR CONSIDERATION

1. Are you hesitant about taking your loved one to the doctor because the symptoms you see don't seem that bad? Please consider the ramifications of not getting an accurate, early diagnosis:

    ¤   Your loved one doesn't get the help they need.
    ¤   Your loved one may miss the opportunity for any last-minute estate planning; that can mean a lot of extra stress on you later if there's no plan in place for their care.

2. What legitimate care options are available to me if my loved one truly does have dementia?

---

34. Mayo Clinic Staff Writer, "Diagnosing Alzheimer's."
35. "Dementia Diagnosis," Mayo Clinic, Mayo Foundation for Medical Education and Research (MFMER), accessed February 2022, mayoclinic.org/diseases-conditions/dementia/diagnosis-treatment/drc-20352019

CHAPTER 3

FINANCIAL CONSIDERATIONS

I n this chapter we will,

- Examine the choices and costs of long-term care
- Define the difference between Medicare and Medicaid
- Discuss Medicaid eligibility
- Review options when only one spouse needs long-term care

More than any other aspect of elder care, the area of financial preparation seems to be the most difficult to grasp. One reason is because the laws which govern Medicare and Medicaid vary from state to state; they are also subject to frequent change. As you will see, a family's "ideal" care solution may not be the most practical one, financially speaking. So, what is the best care solution for your loved one, and how much will it cost?

BUT WE'RE NOT BUYING THE WHOLE FACILITY...

Audrey explained that [my grandparents'] out-of-pocket monthly payments would be several hundred dollars per person, even with insurance helping out. It wouldn't take long for their money to disappear at that rate....

**Excerpt from *Goodnight, Sweet: A Caregiver's Long Goodbye*
Chapter 14: "Vivian"**

The issue of long-term care is not a new one; as the population continues to live longer, options for the health and well-being of the elderly have been steadily undergoing changes. The societal goal is to facilitate a balance between the amount of care required and the quality of life experienced, and there are a multitude of choices available ranging in price from, "My goodness, that's expensive," all the way up to, "Wow—who can afford *that?*" In the broadest sense, the available options include caring for your family member in your home, moving them into an assisted living community, or placing them in a nursing home.

Home Care

Keeping an elderly loved one in your own home is a wonderful plan, but it must be viewed realistically. If you are employed, having to take your loved one back and forth to doctors will probably mean lost time from your job; with very few exceptions, employers have not traditionally been very supportive when the caregiving role intersects with professional responsibilities. Caregiver.org reports that seventy percent of caregivers suffer work-related difficulties because of their dual roles (caregiver vs. company employee).[36] Lost time from work can mean lost wages, and that's a daunting reality for the average caregiver, considering that in 2021 it was reported by *AARP* that dementia caregivers spent more than $7,000 annually in out-of-pocket expenses relating to their caregiving roles.[37]

Then there is the question of your own ability to handle medical situations. By the time my grandparents were at the end of their lives in 1999, the amount of medical care they each required went well beyond anything I was trained to do. Today there are many resources available that make caring for your elderly loved one at home a little easier. A simple internet search for home health care agencies instantly reveals a multitude of choices for medical services which come directly into your home, and many of them are covered by Medicare. You can also find a plethora of adult day care centers in your local area at an average national cost of $74/day.[38] In addition, there is the option to hire a private nurse to help with your loved one's care, and that cost averages out to just over $24/hour, an amount which can go up if the nurse has specialized skills or more advanced training.[39]

You must also consider your season of life: Are you married? Do you have children? Are they toddlers, teens, or twenty-somethings? How will keeping an aging loved one in your home affect everyone else who lives there? And perhaps most important: as your loved one continues to age, are you prepared for their care to take more and more of your time and effort?

---

36. "Caregiver Statistics: Work and Caregiving," Family Caregiver Alliance, accessed February 2022, caregiver.org/resource/caregiver-statistics-work-and-caregiving/

37. Nancy Kerr, "Family Caregivers Spend More than $7,200 a Year on Out-of-Pocket Costs," AARP, June 29, 2021, aarp.org/caregiving/financial-legal/info-2021/high-out-of-pocket-costs/?cmp=RDRCT-867fa361-20211014

38. Scott Witt, Jeff Hoyt, "Adult Day Care Costs," SeniorLiving.org, Centerfield Media Company, updated March 7, 2022 , seniorliving.org/adult-day-care/costs/

39. "Average Nurse Private Duty Hourly Pay," PayScale, Inc., accessed February 2022, payscale.com/research/US/Job=Nurse_Private_Duty/Hourly_Rate

The fact is that while in-home care generally means better conditions for the elderly, it can impose an overwhelming burden on the caregiver. According to the Alzheimer's Association's *2019 Alzheimer's Disease Facts and Figures,* there is a physical and emotional impact to dementia caregiving which resulted in $11.8 billion in *caregiver* health care costs in 2018.[40] Even with help coming in multiple times per week, when you commit to provide care for your loved one in your own home you take on a responsibility that is 24/7. To maintain such a commitment means you must be prepared to keep watch over your own health and well-being. Caregivers have a tendency to get so wrapped up in the job of providing care that they often neglect their own needs, and the result is increased caregiver anxiety and depression which can cause a host of medical issues. You must remember the only way to provide quality care for someone else is to make sure you stay on your A-game, and that means taking the necessary time off and looking after your own health.

Assisted Living

For many people who require long-term care, an assisted living community may sound very appealing. In this scenario, due consideration must be given to obtaining long-term care insurance because of the cost involved. According to Genworth's 2020 Cost of Care Survey, the national average for an assisted living one-bedroom unit is $51,600 annually; this breaks down to $4,300 per month.[41]

Unlike traditional health insurance, long-term care insurance is set up to cover long-term services and supports, including care that is both personal and custodial (non-medical assistance with the activities of daily life).[42] According to aboutassistedliving.org, if you have a long-term care insurance policy, it *should* cover assisted living costs.[43] The safety features, nutritional meal preparation, and socialization make assisted living a great option for seniors.

---

40. "2019 Alzheimer's Disease Facts and Figures," Alzheimer's Association, pg. 38, accessed February 2022, alz.org/media/Documents/alzheimers-facts-and-figures-2019-r.pdf

41. "Cost of Care Survey," Genworth, Genworth Financial, Inc., accessed February 2022, genworth.com/aging-and-you/finances/cost-of-care.html

42. "What Is Long-Term Care Insurance?" Administration for Community Living, Administration on Aging, an official U.S. government website managed by the U.S. Department of Health & Human Services, last modified on February 18, 2020, acl.gov/ltc/costs-and-who-pays/what-is-long-term-care-insurance

43. Contributing authors Kelli Wilson, James Conte, Melinda Booher & Carolyn Falconer-Horne, "How Can I Pay for Assisted Living?" AboutAssistedLiving.org, accessed March 2022, aboutassistedliving.org/how-can-i-pay-for-assisted-living

It is noteworthy that many assisted living communities have included in their programs something called **memory care**. These programs provide long-term skilled nursing designed for patients who have memory issues and/or various forms of dementia, including Alzheimer's.[44] Because the treatment in a memory care unit is so much more involved than a regular assisted living community, the costs can be higher. As of 2021, payments required to live in a private room in a memory care unit averaged just over $5,700 per month.[45] Those costs for memory care may or may not be covered by long-term care insurance; it is contingent on the type of coverage a patient has elected to purchase.[46]

Nursing Home

Most people would agree that going into a nursing home would not be a first choice for those requiring long-term care. For my grandparents, however, it was our only reasonable option. Ironically, it's not *only* placement in the home which causes the patient and their family members distress, but it's also the financial requirements; the monthly cost is staggering.

Genworth's 2021 Cost of Care Survey shows the annual national average cost of a nursing home is $108,408 for a private room; a semi-private room comes in only slightly less at $94,896.[47] Many different factors affect the cost of a nursing home, including its location, the size of the facility, the services offered, and the length of a patient's stay. When you consider everything available for every single patient in a nursing home—all utilities, three meals provided daily by a fully staffed kitchen, laundry services, hospital-type beds, a twenty-four-hour medical staff with their equipment, a front office team of medical social workers, and a director and all of their assistants—the cost makes a little more sense; but more often than not the nursing home never feels quite the way "home" felt.

One major concern people have about nursing homes is the sheer number of sub-standard evaluations reported. The news is rife with stories

44. Merritt Whitley, "Assisted Living vs. Memory Care: What's the Difference?" A Place for Mom, July 12, 2021, aplaceformom.com/caregiver-resources/articles/assisted-living-vs-memory-care

45. "What Does Memory Care Cost?" RetirementLiving, RetirementLiving.com LLC, July 9, 2021, retirementliving.com/what-does-memory-care-cost

46. "Long Term Care Insurance; What is Long Term Care Insurance & What Does it Cover?" SeniorCare.com, accessed March 2022, seniorcare.com/assisted-living/resources/ways-to-pay-for-assisted-living/long-term-care-insurance/

47. "Cost of Care Survey," Genworth, Genworth Financial, Inc., accessed March 2022, genworth.com/aging-and-you/finances/cost-of-care.html

which indicate "below average" care in nursing homes on multiple levels. The apprehension felt by family members who are compelled to leave their loved one in that environment can be overwhelming, but there are steps one can take to head off some of the major issues.

When my grandparents had to go into the nursing home, I made sure to cultivate a positive relationship with the people who were responsible for their care—everyone from the office staff to my grandparents' therapists, nurses, and doctors. In addition to my regular Sunday afternoon visits, I would also come and go at odd hours during the week; that way the staff learned they could never tell when I might show up. I was also vigilant to observe details of my grandparents' appearance. I was always on the lookout for any cuts or bruises, signs they hadn't been bathed, or any indications of a lack of proper care.

It is best to thoroughly research any nursing home before agreeing to admit your loved one. Visit the community, talk to the family members of other residents, and ask questions of the staff. In addition, you can use this link to search a particular nursing home by zip code and have a look at their most recent evaluations: *medicare.gov/nursinghomecompare/search.html*.

It will be highly beneficial to both you and your loved one if you take the time at the beginning of the journey and thoroughly check things out. You'll never regret your due diligence.

MEDI-WHAT?

I was angry about my own ignorance of things like Medicare and other forms of insurance for the post sixty-five crowd.

Excerpt from *Goodnight, Sweet: A Caregiver's Long Goodbye*
Chapter 12: "Anger and Guilt"

So how *do* patients manage to pay for it all? That's where *Medicare* and *Medicaid* come in. For clarification, let's make a clear distinction between these two terms which are sometimes used interchangeably by mistake:

- **Medicare** is the federally funded insurance program which provides health care coverage for Americans who are 65+. It DOES NOT cover long-term care.
- **Medicaid** is a federal/state funded health insurance program for low-income individuals and those with disabilities. It DOES cover long-term care.

31

Medicare

People who are 65 and above are eligible for *Medicare*; it is a form of medical insurance fully funded by the federal government. Depending on the type of coverage an individual chooses, it can help seniors pay for doctors' visits, medications, medical procedures, and hospital stays, but **it *does not* cover long-term care.** Many elderly people use Medicare along with a supplemental insurance which can step in and cover costs that go beyond what Medicare will pay for (this is sometimes referred to as **Medigap**); it's sold by private insurance companies.[48] For specific coverage and eligibility information, visit *medicare.gov.*

Medicaid

When a person requires long-term care and has neither the insurance nor the funds to pay for the necessary services out of pocket, they can apply for *Medicaid* from the state in which they live. Medicaid's funding comes from a combination of state and federal dollars,[49] but it's administered by the states.[50] For more specific information about Medicaid and what it covers, visit *medicaid.gov.*

But Can You Prove They Need It?

"[Mr. Meade] was denied on the grounds of insufficient proof of medical necessity," Audrey said.

Excerpt from *Goodnight, Sweet: A Caregiver's Long Goodbye*
Chapter 17: "Financial Responsibilities"

[As we are looking at Medicaid eligibility only in the context of elder care, this book will devote attention exclusively to that area and will not examine Medicaid's provision for low-income individuals or those with disabilities; for more information on those areas, go to *medicaid.gov.*]

There are two specific things that will be assessed in regard to an elderly person's application for Medicaid: **functionality** and **financial means.**[51]

---

48. "What's Medicare Supplement Insurance (Medigap)?" Medicare.gov, accessed March 2022, medicare.gov/supplements-other-insurance/whats-medicare-supplement-insurance-medigap

49. "What is Medicaid?" HealthInsurance.org, accessed March 2022, healthinsurance.org/glossary/medicaid/

50. Created by FindLaw's team of legal writers and editors, "The Difference Between Medicare and Medicaid," FindLaw, Thomson Reuters, June 12, 2018, findlaw.com/healthcare/medicare-medicaid/the-difference-between-medicare-and-medicaid.html

51. "Medicaid Eligibility: 2022 Income, Asset & Care Requirements for Nursing Homes & Long-Term Care," American Council on Aging, last updated December 6, 2021, medicaidplanningassistance.org/medicaid-eligibility/

Functionality

Medicaid will make the determination as to whether or not a person has a need for the level of care provided by a long-term care facility. In other words, does the patient demonstrate a **medical necessity**? After my grandparents' resources had been spent down to the allowable amount, my grandfather's Medicaid application was denied because the accompanying documentation failed to show medical necessity. Just looking at a group of test results in a file didn't convey the true severity of his dementia. In preparing the next Medicaid application, the nursing home's medical social worker gathered every report available on my grandfather's state of mind; meanwhile, I petitioned the doctors who had done earlier examinations on him to write letters clarifying his definite need for long-term care as he was no longer competent to look after his own well-being. The added materials worked, and my grandfather was finally accepted as a Medicaid recipient.

Financial Means

Medicaid representatives will also examine an applicant's complete financial portfolio. There are a number of financial factors involved in determining if an applicant meets Medicaid's stringent requirements for coverage.

In very general terms, Medicaid requires that an applicant's assets be liquified (converted into cash) and spent down so that the applicant has no more than $2,000 (an amount that can vary by state) remaining in their checking account. Assets that would be viewed as needing to be "spent down" include cash, monies held in bank accounts, property other than one's primary residence, 401Ks, mutual funds, stocks, bonds, certificates of deposit, and (sometimes) IRAs that aren't in the payout status.[52]

One important thing to note: if a Medicaid applicant is already receiving Social Security benefits, the applicant (or the individual with Power of Attorney for the applicant) will need to speak to a Medicaid representative to determine how much (if any) Social Security monies may be kept in the applicant's checking account. In my grandparents' case, they were both living in the nursing home with Medicaid footing the bill, so when their Social Security checks were deposited into their bank, I had to write a check to the nursing home for any amount that put them over the $2,000-per-person limit ($4,000 between them). Essentially, it was considered to be payment toward their care.

52. "Spending Down Assets to Become Medicaid Eligible for Nursing Home/Long Term Care," American Council on Aging, last updated December 14, 2021, medicaidplanningassistance.org/medicaid-spend-down/

So the excess money needs to be spent down; but exactly *what* you're allowed to purchase as you "spend down" your loved one's assets can get complicated. From a 50,000-foot overview, your loved one's money can be spent down on anything that helps *them*. For example, if they have debts, their cash can go toward paying off those debts; if there are no pre-paid funeral arrangements, the assets that exceed $2,000 can be used to take care of that need; they can also purchase any medical equipment which is not covered by their insurance.[53] Whatever the money is spent on must be something which takes care of *them*, not another family member or friend.

Sometimes elderly people want to "gift" their money (or some other big-ticket asset like property or a vehicle) to a son or daughter or perhaps to a grandchild or even a close friend. Federal tax law for 2022 states that you can annually give someone up to $16,000 without any penalty tax;[54] but right here let's make a clear distinction: **federal tax law** and **Medicaid regulations**—these are *two totally different things*. When your loved one applies for Medicaid, their assets will be subject to a "look-back period" of five years. If a Medicaid applicant has gifted *any* money or assets to *anyone* for *any* reason during that review of the previous five years, Medicaid can deny approval and compel them to wait until five years after the time of the original gifting before approving the application.

Another concern for Medicaid applicants is whether an applicant's home will be considered an asset which must be "spent down"; in other words, would the home have to be sold and the proceeds spent down before Medicaid would approve their application? In general terms, an applicant's primary residence is considered an exempt asset; it will not be counted when they apply for Medicaid as long as the equity interest in the home falls below $585,000.[55] However, upon the death of the Medicaid recipient, the Medicaid Estate Recovery Program (MERP) may attempt to recoup all or some of their investment. MERP can reach into the proceeds from the sale of the Medicaid recipient's home[56] before any monies are divided among family members as directed by a will. It is advisable to seek the advice of an estate planning attorney who is experienced with Medicaid so that all proper measures are taken to legally protect an inheritance.

---

53. American Council on Aging, "Spending Down Assets."

54. Liz Smith, "Gift Tax Limits: How Much Can You Gift?" SmartAsset, SmartAsset Advisors, LLC, December 31, 2021, smartasset.com/retirement/gift-tax-limits

55. K. Gabriel Heiser, "Can Medicaid Take a Senior's House to Pay Their Nursing Home Bill?" AgingCare.com, accessed March 2022, agingcare.com/Articles/can-medicaid-take-your-house-147803.htm

56. Heiser, "Can Medicaid Take a Senior's House?"

A House Divided

The doctors are telling me that Grandpa is doing better than Grandma....

Excerpt from *Goodnight, Sweet: A Caregiver's Long Goodbye*
Chapter 11: "Evidence and Denial"

Sadly, it's not uncommon for one spouse to receive a diagnosis that requires a far greater level of care than the other spouse, and frequently the healthier spouse is not able to meet that care need. If the couple has the financial means, they can move together into an assisted living community; but generally speaking, Medicaid won't cover that cost.

If the couple cannot afford the cost of assisted living, the next step is to consider nursing home care which can be covered by Medicaid. The spouse in need can apply for Medicaid, but where does that leave the healthy spouse—the one still living in the couple's shared home—and what about their shared assets?

In 1988, Congress made provisions for the **community spouse**—the healthier spouse who is still living in the community, *not* in the nursing home. To keep the community spouse from becoming impoverished if the unhealthy spouse has to go into a nursing home utilizing Medicaid, there is a **minimum monthly maintenance needs allowance** (MMMNA) as well as a **monthly housing allowance**. The MMMNA can vary by state, but the range for 2019 is generally between $2,000 and $3,000 monthly,[57] with an additional $600–700 (again, depending on the state) allocated for the monthly housing allowance. Thanks to Medicaid's spousal impoverishment provision, "A certain amount of the couple's combined resources is protected for the community spouse."[58] The amount of countable assets the community spouse is allowed to keep without disqualifying the Medicaid applicant is known as the **Community Spouse Resource Allowance** (CSRA).

The CSRA is determined by both federal and state rules. It is advisable to speak with a Medicaid representative and/or an estate planning attorney who is well-versed in Medicaid regulations to ensure that assets are being handled correctly.

---

57. "2022 SSI and Spousal Impoverishment Standards," PDF, benefits.com/news/cms-ssi-and-spousal-impoverishment-standards

58. "Spousal Impoverishment," Medicaid.gov, Access date, March 2022, https://www.medicaid.gov/medicaid/eligibility/spousal-impoverishment/index.html

QUESTIONS FOR CONSIDERATION

1. Realistically, what long-term option will provide your loved one the best possible care, considering both financial and relational dynamics?

2. With the understanding that the financial decisions you make now can affect your ability to receive governmental financial aid in the future, if you or your loved one were to require long-term care, what can you do today to ensure that an application for Medicaid would not be denied?

3. Do you have a working knowledge of your loved one's financial portfolio?
   - Do you know where they bank?
   - What kind of retirement accounts do they have?
   - What are the sources of all current income (Social Security, investments, etc.)?
   - How much do those monthly deposits total?
   - Can you access all of your loved one's accounts?

CHAPTER 4

FAMILY RELATIONSHIPS

I n this chapter we will,
- Examine pre-planning as a way to reduce conflict
- Look at the role of a mediator
- Discuss having negative feelings toward the one needing care
- Explore the option of forgiveness

Being a caregiver for the dementia patient (or, for that matter, any patient) is a difficult role even when all the right steps have been taken ahead of time. Having the correct legal documentation, medical help, and financial preparations in place is sure to relieve a lot of caregiver stress, but there is one area that is as uniquely unpredictable as any dementia symptom ever encountered: the dynamic of relationships between family members—particularly in the throes of a family crisis.

WHAT GIVES YOU THE RIGHT TO SAY WHAT HAPPENS?

> *"So, you have power of attorney,"* [Shirley] said...."*I guess you're also the executor of the estate?"*
>
> **Excerpt from *Goodnight, Sweet: A Caregiver's Long Goodbye***
> **Chapter 20: "Confrontation"**

If there's one single point that should motivate you to finalize your own estate plan, it's knowing that right now you have the opportunity to name your own caregiver. Trouble among family members may be significantly reduced by your personal designation of someone who can act with authority on your behalf in the event you become incapacitated. In the long run, less in-fighting among relatives can translate to better care for you. For much the same reason, it is equally important that we aid our elderly loved ones in establishing their own estate plan before something should occur that would prevent them from doing so.

Choosing a person to act as your agent may seem like an impossible task. How do you decide who will bear all that responsibility? Ideally you want a person you trust, someone with whom you have a good relationship and who has the ability to manage a range of issues such as finances, medical decisions, and communication with family members.

As I mentioned in chapter one, it may be beneficial to consider splitting up the necessary duties—depending on the strengths and weaknesses of the individuals involved. For example, if there are two adult children and one of them is particularly good with money, it might be wise to appoint that one to serve with a financial power of attorney. Maybe one is good at handling the medical side of things, so they might do well with the medical power of attorney—one who can competently make any necessary medical decisions. In families where there are multiple siblings, make every effort to ensure the caregiving duties are divided in a balanced way so people will feel neither slighted nor overburdened.

Pre-appointing one's own choice(s) for future care may also help secure the legal footing of the person designated. In my case, I had two half-brothers who had very little contact with our grandparents; therefore, when it came time for our grandparents to appoint someone to serve them with durable power of attorney, I was an obvious choice because of our good and well-established relationship. Neither of my half-brothers ever attempted any legal maneuver to remove me from my appointed position, but even if they had tried, they would have been hard-pressed to present a valid reason for doing so. The POA documents naming me as the Meades' appointed agent had been on file with their attorney for five years prior to the documents' activations, and I made sure that my handling of everything from their medical care to their finances was completely transparent. My grandparents' pre-planning was instrumental in establishing my position, virtually ensuring that my care for them wouldn't be disrupted by legal challenges.

Now at this point you might be thinking that if I didn't have any legal challenges to my authority to act for my grandparents, then how qualified am I to write a chapter on the caregiver's exasperation with extended family members? Well, I may not have been challenged *legally*, but I certainly had my share of people who weighed in frequently and vividly on a wide range of subjects associated with my care of Edward and Clara Meade. Some were very kind and supportive while others wanted to complain or give advice. The "advisors" were usually family members who cloaked themselves with a mantle of concern, and they always wanted to know the same basic things:

One: *What was I ultimately going to do with them?*

Two: *Was there a will?*

(And the rarely spoken but always clearly implied:)

Three: *Who was in line for the inheritance?*

And then there were the folks in the "I just thought you should know" category. A distant cousin once read me the riot act because I was actually allowing my grandparents to live in a community where they had to *share a bathroom* with the resident in the next room. Another time a phlebotomist looked me straight in my face and told me that unless I had a death-wish for my grandparents, I should immediately move them out of Waverly Nursing Home because the staff there was so bad. And one of the most bizarre queries came courtesy of a relative who had more concern for Grandma's *pillowcases*—yes, I'm serious—than she had for Grandma herself. She called me and asked in a breathy, anxious voice if I'd secured them. Oh yes, I've dealt with my share of outlandish comments, questions, and suggestions.

At the end of the day, I knew I was doing the best I could with the resources available to me. One of the greatest pieces of wisdom I have to offer caregivers is this: **Do the best you can for your loved one.** Remember, they entrusted *you* with their care, so do not let yourself be pulled down by complainers and naysayers who only want to run their mouths to nit-pick rather than offer any real help. When you know you're doing all you can, you deserve the peace of mind that comes with letting their criticism just roll off.

SLEEPING VOLCANOS

"Maybe [my half-brothers and their mother] won't be disagreeable over all this," I speculated.

"They ought to be thrilled that it's you in the decision-making hot seat and not them," Chris said firmly.

Excerpt from *Goodnight, Sweet: A Caregiver's Long Goodbye*
Chapter 19: "Contact"

When a loved one transitions from "possibly needing care" into the "definitely needs care" phase, the journey for their caregiver is one filled with uncertainty, self-doubt, and emotional pain—and those are the feelings of the designated agent who faces *no challenge* from other family members. But real-life families don't come packaged like the ones found in fiction; tempers can flare among even the most loving relatives. Disagreement often ensues as the discussion of what to do with mother or father, aunt, uncle, or grandparent gets underway. Situations can get particularly dicey if there's been "bad blood" between family members. Bitter feelings can smolder just below the surface for years, waiting for the right situation to set off an eruption that rivals Vesuvius.

Sometimes an adult son or daughter becomes jealous because their parent has chosen one of their siblings over them to provide care. This often results in anger toward both the parent and the chosen sibling. Another common situation that can stir up trouble is when the sibling living in closest proximity to the parent is chosen to be the caregiver by default. That caregiver tends to experience the feeling of having no choice in the matter which leads to resentment of not only their parent but also the sibling who "escaped" the caregiver role.

Situations like these can lead to shattered family relationships, often leaving individuals so entrenched in their positions they won't even speak to each other. And when you factor in one sibling having complete control over Mom or Dad's money—as well as the autonomy to make all of their medical decisions—you have the ingredients for a bona fide family feud.

Initially, deadlocked family members might try asking the family attorney for help; matters of contention can be discussed on neutral ground in the attorney's office. Consideration might also be given to a church counselor or a professional therapist for the same reason: neutral ground.

In the event these options aren't able to reverse the escalation of tensions, it may be necessary to ask a professional mediator for help. A professional mediator is someone who is trained to act as a go-between; they are personally uninvolved in the situation and can therefore listen to both sides without bias. They tend to see the issues more clearly and therefore may be able to facilitate a satisfactory resolution to the conflict. The mediator strives to help each party see previously unthought-of ways to solve the problems that face them, and, in the end, successful mediation could save the family a costly legal battle.[59] A simple internet search of "family mediation" can yield a variety of professionals, both on the national level and in your local area.

"I DON'T CARE WHAT HAPPENS TO YOU!"

I was absolutely refusing to admit that I was horribly angry about being saddled with the tremendous responsibility and, yes, the burden of caring for Grandma and Grandpa. Having to actually admit that I saw it as a burden was more than I was ready to deal with.

**Excerpt from *Goodnight, Sweet: A Caregiver's Long Goodbye*
Chapter 12: "Anger and Guilt"**

59. Christina Ianzito, "How to Choose an Elder Mediator," AARP, February 6, 2017, aarp.org/caregiving/financial-legal/info-2017/how-to-choose-caregiver-mediator.html

What if the bitter feelings aren't between the family members arguing over the caregiver role? What if the caregiver is holding resentment, hostility, or unforgiveness against the one who needs care? This is not an uncommon situation because, as we acknowledged in the previous section, families don't always play nice. In my own case, I did have to work through an initial onslaught of anger as I realized *why* the overwhelming responsibility to care for my grandparents fell on me alone: because their son (my biological father) was nowhere to be found. I was able to work with relative speed through my negative feelings once I understood they were based on my resentment of their son's willful absence rather than some kind of actual malice toward Grandma and Grandpa. Deep down I truly loved *them*, and I knew that my care for them was a genuine reciprocation of the love and affection they'd always shown me.

But there are situations where bitterness and unforgiveness seem to be the order of the day. Parents who played favorites among their children or those who were very authoritarian and unyielding can wind up with a younger generation who wants nothing but miles between themselves and the offending parent. Those who had a hard time expressing anything positive during their child's formative years may discover their now adult son or daughter is filled with resentment for their lack of parental affirmation. The resulting animosity can harden into an attitude that says, "I'm never going to forgive you—get *away* from me!" For clarity, allow me to borrow from the familiar world of fiction: consider the resentment—the sheer teeth-clenching, blood-boiling anger—that Cinderella might feel if she was tapped to serve as her step-mother's caregiver. I think that given her step-mother's behavior, Cinderella would feel little, *if any*, motivation to make sure her step-mother received proper care.

The tragedy here is that sooner or later the emotionally wounded adult might have to face a situation where their cold, harsh, demanding parent can no longer manage on their own. Adding insult to injury, the abrasive parent may even express that the "child" they raised owes them a debt of gratitude and therefore has a duty—a moral obligation—to help their aging parent. The adult son or daughter may go ahead and shoulder the responsibility, but many times they're doing so because they feel trapped, and they wonder if there's not *some* way they can just walk out and never have to look back.

IF I FORGIVE YOU…

[The Holy Spirit] entered into the dark place with me.…He led me back into the light with gentle ease, and His willingness to

41

forgive me became my willingness to take my hands off [Shirley's] proverbial throat.

**Excerpt from *Goodnight, Sweet: A Caregiver's Long Goodbye*
Chapter 19: "Contact"**

If someone is holding offense and unforgiveness toward another person—like we just examined in the previous section—that offense and unforgiveness is only hurting the one holding it, *not* the one against whom it's held. This is such a difficult area because when we're angry or hurt the *last* thing we want to do is let it go. We tend to want revenge, *to see them pay* for what they've done; but this is bad news for the one who won't forgive. Studies abound which show how forgiveness is extremely beneficial to *one's own* health; advantages include lowering the risk of heart attack, improving cholesterol levels and sleep, as well as reducing pain, blood pressure, anxiety, depression, and stress.[60]

Let me clarify that I am not an expert in psychology or human behavior, but I've certainly had experience with being offended and hurt by the choices of other people. For that reason, I would like to take at least a cursory look at the issues of offense and forgiveness, examining them from the perspective of my own personal involvement peppered with a goodly amount of research.

Sometimes we are given the impression that forgiveness is supposed to happen in a snap of the fingers; one, two, three—and it's done! But my own experience tells me this simply is not so. The greater the violation, the more difficult true forgiveness can be. Even after saying that I forgive the offense, the memory of it and the feelings that memory stirs up are often just below the surface, ready to pop out at any moment. And the more recent the event, the more easily the memories are stirred. Frequency and duration of the offense also play an important role in determining the level of difficulty you may experience as you set your mind to genuinely forgive someone.

The difficulty of forgiveness can also depend on the degree of the offense; little issues may be resolved fairly quickly, while deep hurts brought on by the perception of great violation can take quite a while to heal. It can be a difficult task, one that must be accurately identified as a process rather than simply saying the words, "Oh, OK, I'll forgive you!"

The process of true forgiveness has often required that I keep going to God over and over again to reiterate that I forgive my offender and their offense until it's all settled in my mind. Offenses may be real, or they may

---

60. "Forgiveness: Your Health Depends on It," Johns Hopkins Medicine, The Johns Hopkins University, The Johns Hopkins Hospital, and Johns Hopkins Health System, accessed March 2022, hopkinsmedicine.org/health/wellness-and-prevention/forgiveness-your-health-depends-on-it

only be *perceived* as real. Sometimes events occur in which the offender has no idea they've done something to "offend" the other person. The issue is one of perception; if a person *perceives* an offense, whether anything was meant by it or not, that person will behave as if the offense is real—carrying *real* unforgiveness and *real* bitterness.

I can illustrate what I mean by describing the process the Holy Spirit took me through to resolve feelings of deep anger directed at Ray Meade, my biological father. As I described in chapter two of *Goodnight, Sweet: A Caregiver's Long Goodbye*, Ray had committed bigamy, leaving my mother and me to fend for ourselves. After being brought to account for what he'd done and subsequently being divorced from my mother, Ray wanted absolutely nothing to do with me. His rejection of me left a deep gash in my emotions, and I carried the wound as if it was something I'd never be free of; I *believed* if my own biological father didn't want me then I must not be worth wanting. My assumption from the start was that *I* was the problem.

As a result, I'd grown up with massive trust issues and horribly low self-esteem. Even though I had spent a great deal of time in the counselor's chair, I never really understood the root of the issue which was that the wounds I carried were built on lies and false conclusions.

But Jesus wanted to set me free from those bitter wounds and that crippling resentment. In John 14:6, He said, "I am the way and *the truth* and the life." Jesus wanted me to understand *the truth* of what had happened during the months that followed my birth, so one evening, late into the overnight hours, He allowed me to have a profound and unusual experience.

I had been sleeping soundly when I suddenly came to, and as I laid there wide awake, the Holy Spirit began to stir my thoughts about Ray. As He began to probe, I sensed Him asking me to consider what I believed "the truth" was about Ray's abandonment. All my life I had truly believed that the timing of Ray leaving my mother had to do with the fact that I had been born *and* that I was a girl; I had believed he was so thoroughly disappointed in me that he just walked out. Why else would he have stayed with my mother for five years before I was born only to leave when I was not even two months old? What had changed? Obviously, it was my birth!

But the Holy Spirit began to pull back the curtain, allowing me to clearly understand what had actually happened. *The truth* was that Ray had had a sordid history of cheating on my mother throughout their five-year marriage prior to my birth. *The truth* was that something had changed all right—but it wasn't me being born; it was that one of Ray's many indiscretions had led to an unexpected pregnancy. It may sound ridiculous, but I'd never looked at the timeline that closely, so it was like a brand-new revelation to me—one that let me off the proverbial hook. It turned out that I *wasn't* the issue after all; I had *never* been the issue. The issue had always been the way Ray regarded everyone in his life. He was self-absorbed, and he only looked at what was good for himself, never considering how his actions might affect other people. He treated everyone like play things; when he got tired of one, he merely discarded it in favor of another. In the end he not only discarded me but also my mother, his parents, and eventually his second wife and their two sons—and these are only the ones I know of!

When all was said and done, yes, Ray had still rejected me. He'd still abandoned me; those *facts* didn't change. What had changed was my understanding—my *perception*. I began to comprehend that my birth wasn't the catalyst for Ray to walk out the way he did. My new information—*the truth*—was instrumental in bringing me to a place where I was able to let go of my anger and hurt. The truth allowed me to see that his leaving wasn't my fault; I wasn't guilty of anything! Finally, I was free to pray for Ray, asking God to work in his heart. And by letting go—by choosing to forgive Ray—I let myself experience freedom from the bitterness and resentment I'd lived with for years. Once I chose to let go of the false perception, I was actually open to receive the love that Jesus had had for me all along.

I want to be clear here: your hurts are real, and your feelings are valid; but I promise you the love Jesus has for you is deeper than those hurts, and I'm telling you that I believe He truly can heal your wounds. I know because He healed mine—I've experienced it for myself.

QUESTIONS FOR CONSIDERATION

1. As the primary caregiver, are you prepared to stand your ground when you know you're doing the best thing possible for your loved one, even if other family members are criticizing your actions?

2. Are you open to listen to the suggestions of others and implement them if they can make things better for the one who requires care?

3. Is it possible for you to "clear the air" with your loved one regarding any bitter feelings you may have toward them? Can you think far enough ahead to imagine how you'd feel if something happened to them before you were able to do that?

CHAPTER 5

SAFETY

In this chapter we will,

- Identify secure mobility aids
- Examine the safety of elders continuing to drive
- Discuss keeping the dementia patient protected in their environment
- Consider when a long-term care community might be best

One of the greatest sources of concern for any caregiver is the issue of safety. As people age, their reaction times can diminish, and their legs or feet may become unsteady; a once definitive stride might even start looking more like a shuffle. Additionally, there may be problems with balance and concerns about brittle bones. Any of these natural signs of aging could eventually lead to compromised safety for our senior adults. With dementia patients, caregivers have additional safety concerns such as what can happen if the patient forgets they left water running in a sink or bathtub. Or what if they randomly turn on a stove or an oven then walk out of the kitchen and forget about it? At any given time, caregivers have a multitude of things vying for their attention, but safety for the one needing care is always at the top of the list.

WHEN "UPWARDLY MOBILE" MEANS GETTING UP OUT OF A CHAIR

The nursing [home] supervisor told me Grandma had had a very bad fall, forcefully hitting the back of her head against the floor.

Excerpt from *Goodnight, Sweet: A Caregiver's Long Goodbye*
Chapter 23: "Hello, Sweet"

One of the greatest health concerns seniors face is the risk of falling. It is actually one of the most common ways an elderly person sustains an injury.[61]

---

61. "Injury Prevention & Control," Centers for Disease Control and Prevention, U.S. Department of Health & Human Services, accessed March 2022, cdc.gov/injury/features/older-adult-falls/index.html#:~:text=Falls%20and%20motor%20vehicle%20crashes,%2C%20mobile%2C%20and%20independent%20tomorrow

During the time I was caring for my grandparents, Grandma had two falls; one was shortly before she left her home in 1997, and the other was in the nursing home two weeks before her death in 1999. Whether your senior is at home or in a long-term care community, you need to be aware of any mobility issues because they *are* such a major safety concern. Limited mobility in seniors can be caused by a number of things, including the following:

- **Injuries**: Slips and trips can take a greater toll on elderly people because bones and muscles tend to weaken with age.
- **Osteoarthritis**: Cartilage that cushions the joints wears down with age, so joints become inflamed, resulting in swelling, stiffness, and pain.
- **Neuropathy**: Seniors with this condition may have muscle weakness, cramps, and muted reflexes, all of which can make walking difficult.
- **Heart conditions**: Seniors with cardiovascular issues are more prone to being dizzy, lightheaded, and short of breath. These difficulties can cause them to be less active which leaves them less flexible and therefore less mobile.

It's important for caregivers to take every necessary precaution to avoid problems from the start.

Have a "Falls Risk Assessment" Done

A **Falls Risk Assessment** is an evaluation conducted in the office of your loved one's physician; it's designed to help determine how likely it is that a patient will fall.

- The clinician will ask questions like, "Have you had a fall during the last year?" or "Do you feel unsteady when you stand or walk?"
- The assessment will also take the patient through a series of simple movements to test their strength, balance, and gait (the way they walk).

If your loved one's physician determines there is an increased risk of falling, they may be able to recommend strategies to prevent falls thereby reducing the chance of injury.[62]

---

62. "Fall Risk Assessment," MedlinePlus, National Library of Medicine, U.S. Department of Health and Human Services, National Institutes of Health, Last updated September 13, 2021, medlineplus.gov/lab-tests/fall-risk-assessment/#:~:text=A%20fall%20risk%20assessment%20is,reduce%20the%20chance%20of%20injury

Cane vs. Walker[63]

A walking aid might be helpful, but determining which one to use will depend on what type of support is needed. If there is weakness or mild pain on one side in a hip, knee, or foot, a **cane** can provide support by reducing the weight on the side with the trouble. Remember,

- The cane should be held in the hand *opposite* the weak/painful side.
- The cane should move at the same time as the weak/painful side.
- On the stairs, the good leg should go first followed by the weak/painful leg and the cane.[64]

Canes are available in a variety of handle shapes, heights, and base types; your physician should be able to determine what type of cane will be the most helpful to your loved one.

If there is pain/weakness on both sides of the body, a **walker** (a frame with handles and legs that needs to be picked up to move) or a **rollator** (a frame which has wheels and can be pushed) will provide a better base of support.

- Walkers are usually made from aluminum so they are lightweight and can be moved easily.
- Walkers usually have rubber caps on the legs to make them more stable.[65]
- Rollators (sometimes referred to as "wheeled walkers") may be made from aluminum or steel, and they may come with two, three, or even four wheels, depending on the type of support that's needed; they have handlebars, and most have a built-in seat.[66]
- Rollators come equipped with brakes.

  - **Loop-lock brakes**, located under the handlebars: to engage, the user will squeeze both loops.
  - **Hand brakes**: these are manufactured as a single brake to be used with one hand, or like a bicycle with brakes on both handles; the user will squeeze the hand brake toward the handle to stop the motion.

63. Barbara Stepko, "Choosing a Walker or Cane," AARP, March 6, 2020, aarp.org/health/healthy-living/info-2020/walkers-canes.html

64. Am Fam Physician, "How to Use Canes and Walkers," American Family Physician, American Academy of Family Physicians, June 15, 2021, aafp.org/afp/2021/0615/p737-s1.html

65. Brian Carmody, "The Features of Different Walkers," Fact checked by Marley Hall, VeryWellHealth, Dotdash Media, Inc., March 2, 2020, verywellhealth.com/walker-or-rollator-2318325

66. Brian Carmody, "How a Rollator Differs from a Walker," Medically reviewed by Isaac O. Opole, MD, PhD, Fact checked by Marley Hall, VeryWellHealth.com, Dotdash Media, Inc., updated December 6, 2020, verywellhealth.com/rollator-or-walker-2318324

    ¤   **Push-down brakes** which are weight-activated: they are engaged by downward pressure on the handles.[67]

The decision of whether to get a walker or a rollator will depend largely on the upper body strength of the patient; your physician should be able to determine what equipment will be the most helpful to your loved one.

Walkers and rollators can often be purchased in your local pharmacy if you pay out of pocket. **Medicare Part B** may cover walkers and rollators as **durable medical equipment** (DME), but the item must be deemed medically necessary and prescribed by your physician or other treating provider for in-home use.[68]

Wheelchair vs. Scooter

Some patients have mobility issues that are so profound they are unable to stand or walk at all. In this case, secure movement may require an option where the individual can sit comfortably and roll to their destination.

There are a number of different types of **wheelchairs** available, some of which are highly specialized such as airplane wheelchairs; beach wheelchairs; electric, manual, sports, and transport wheelchairs—just to name a few.[69] If your loved one has a temporary mobility issue (like an injury from which they will recover) and they have good upper body strength, a lightweight manual wheelchair would probably work. For a senior who needs the chair for a longer term, a powered chair might be better.[70] Allow your loved one's physician to give you direction on which choice will work best.

Another option to discuss with the doctor might be the use of a **mobility scooter**. Unlike motorized wheelchairs which can be operated using a joystick (ideal for the person with little or no upper body strength), scooters have a tiller and handle bars—much like a bicycle—and they may have three or four wheels, depending on the needs of the individual using it. Three-wheel scooters are easier to maneuver in small spaces, but the four-wheel scooters provide a wider wheel base and therefore tend

67. "Where Are the Brakes on These Rollators?" JustWalkers.com, accessed March 2022, justwalkers.com/blogs/mobility-blog/wheres-the-brakes-rollators#:~:text=Push%2Ddown%20 brakes%20are%20brakes,a%20less%20stable%20walking%20aid

68. "Walkers: Your Costs in Original Medicare," Medicare.gov, U.S. Center for Medicare and Medicaid Services, accessed March 2022, medicare.gov/coverage/walkers

69. Margaret Sellars, "Different Types of Wheelchairs Available (& Finding the Right Kind)," Mobility Deck, MobilityDeck, accessed March 2022, mobilitydeck.com/ types-of-wheelchairs/#Types_of_Wheelchairs_for_Seniors

70. "Best Wheelchair for Elderly Review 2022," Chair Institute, An Elite Cafe-media Home/DIY Publisher, accessed March 2022, chairinstitute.com/best-wheelchair-for-elderly/

to be more stable—and they can bear a weight of up to five hundred pounds.[71]

Cost is one reason you may want to consider a scooter over a wheelchair; scooters can range in price anywhere from $1,000 up to $5,000, whereas the cost of an enhanced electric wheelchair can go as high as $15,000.[72]

Medicare Part B may cover the cost of a wheelchair or a scooter, considering the vehicle to be durable medical equipment. The caveat is that in addition to the patient's physician submitting a written order stating the medical need for the wheelchair or scooter, there is a pre-determined list of conditions which the patient must also meet.[73] For more detailed information, please visit *www.medicare.gov.*

ROAD TRIP

[Grandpa] said, "Now get me [my] car."

"Grandpa," I hesitated, not really sure what to say to him as he was growing more and more demanding. "I promise you don't need that car."

In one quick, unexpected action, Grandpa violently grabbed my arm and shook me with a hard jerk. "Where is it?" he demanded angrily....I'd never heard such rage in his voice.

Excerpt from *Goodnight, Sweet: A Caregiver's Long Goodbye*
Chapter 13: "Failure"

If your elderly loved one starts showing signs of impaired vision and/or hearing, a slower reaction time, a limited range of motion, or cognition issues, it may be time to talk about them giving up the driver's seat. According to the Centers for Disease Control and Prevention (CDC), drivers who are aged 75 years and up have a higher crash death rate than middle-aged drivers between the ages of 35 and 54;[74] even so, this is one of the most difficult conversations any caregiver will ever have with their loved one.

An individual's ability to drive is a hallmark of independence, so the mere suggestion that it may be time to stop driving can sound to elderly

---

71. "Mobility Scooters," Karman, Karman Healthcare, Inc., accessed March 2022, karmanhealthcare.com/deciding-between-electric-scooter-and-power-wheelchair/

72. Karman, "Mobility Scooters."

73. "Medicare's Wheelchair & Scooter Benefit," Centers for Medicare & Medicaid Services, Department of Health & Human Services, revised October 2019, medicare.gov/Pubs/pdf/11046-Medicare-Wheelchair-Scooter.pdf

74. "Transportation Safety: Older Adult Drivers," Centers for Disease Control and Prevention, U.S. Department of Health & Human Services, accessed March 2022, cdc.gov/transportationsafety/older_adult_drivers/index.html?CDC_AA_refVal=https%3A%2F%2Fwww.cdc.gov%2Fmotorvehiclesafety%2Folder_adult_drivers%2Findex.html

ears like a hostile takeover by the younger generation. The Mayo Clinic offers a few suggestions to help caregivers get the conversation started. They advise that you begin the discussion as soon as possible following a dementia diagnosis, and they recommend involving the doctor.

- Rather than the caregiver autonomously making the decision about their loved one's driving, allow the person with dementia to be involved in the discussion and planning process.
- Begin by talking about their safety and the safety of other drivers.
- Make an appeal to their sense of responsibility.
- And remember, it's imperative for caregivers to be aware of their loved one's feelings regarding this change in driving status.[75]

It's important for you to remain vigilant regarding your elderly loved ones who still drive. According to the National Institutes of Health[76] and AARP,[77] there are a number of specific warning signs which may indicate it's time to take away their keys:

- Have they been involved in multiple vehicle crashes or "near misses" and/or turned up with new dents in the car?
- Have there been comments from neighbors or friends about their driving?
- Do they have any health issues that might affect driving ability?
- Do they confuse the brake and gas pedals?
- Are they driving too slow or too fast consistently?
- Have they gotten lost on familiar roads?
- Do they run red lights or stop signs?
- Do they use (or change) lanes improperly?

The difficulty here is that there is no set age when driving "becomes" impaired; the ability to drive safely is affected by many things. In addition to physical changes that can occur as people age, some medications taken by our elderly loved ones can impede driving ability by contributing to feelings of drowsiness or lightheadedness. Staying alert to your loved one's physical conditions and current medications is paramount for their safety as well as that of other drivers.

75. Dana Sparks, "Alzheimer's and Dementia: When to Stop Driving," Mayo Clinic News Network, Mayo Clinic, November 12, 2019, newsnetwork.mayoclinic.org/discussion/alzheimers-and-dementia-when-to-stop-driving/

76. "National Institute on Aging: Older Drivers," U.S. Department of Health & Human Services, accessed March 2022, nia.nih.gov/health/older-drivers

77. Stacey Colino, "Is it Time for Your Loved One to Retire from Driving?" AARP, updated October 21, 2021, aarp.org/caregiving/basics/info-2019/is-it-time-to-stop-driving.html

Get a Professional Driving Assessment[78]

Just like taking your loved one to their physician for an annual checkup, you may consider having their road skills evaluated through a professional driving assessment. These clinical assessments are conducted by trained specialists who can shed light on a driver's true level of ability. The results of the assessment may clarify...

- If your loved one is perfectly fit to drive without any restrictions
- Whether or not your loved one could use some extra training
- Or that your loved one is no longer safe to drive a vehicle

There are two main categories of driving assessments:

- *Driving skills evaluation:* an in-car evaluation of driving abilities and (if necessary) recommendations about additional driver's training
- *Clinical driving assessment:* used to find any underlying medical causes which may affect safe driving and recommendations to address those issues

The clinical driving assessment will include the following:

- A review of the driver's personal medical history and a cognitive assessment
- An on-road assessment to see if traffic rules are being obeyed as well as observing strategies used to compensate for any impairment
- Treatment and intervention like adaptive driving instruction (helping drivers reacquire their skills after a change in their physical or mental condition[79])

The cost of a professional driving assessment typically ranges between $200 and $400 with an added cost for additional driver training. The American Occupational Therapy Association (AOTA) has put together a nationwide database of driving programs and specialists. Visit *myaota.aota.org/driver_search/index.aspx/index.aspx* for more information on this program.

BUT IS IT DEMENTIA-PROOF?

I knew that here *they would be safe.*

Excerpt from *Goodnight, Sweet: A Caregiver's Long Goodbye*
Chapter 14: "Vivian"

78. "Evaluate Your Driving Ability," AAA Exchange, AAA, accessed March 2022, exchange.aaa.com/safety/senior-driver-safety-mobility/evaluate-your-driving-ability/

79. "Adaptive Driving," BaylorScott&White Institute for Rehabilitation, accessed March 2022, bswrehab.com/levels-of-care/outpatient-therapy/therapy-services/adaptivedriving/

For the average person, safety in the home is a top priority at any age. It is not uncommon for expectant parents to "baby proof" their home, and there are lots of people who utilize home security systems—all in the name of protecting themselves and their loved ones from possible harm. The common theme is trying to anticipate potential dangers and actively looking to stop them *before* something bad can happen.

In the same way, caregivers must ensure that their elderly loved one's environment is free from things that could cause them harm. This is not as easy as it may sound because caring for a dementia patient is such a "fluid" situation—the changes may be fast or slow, but their occurrence is certain.

Home Safety Evaluation[80]

You can request that your loved one's physician order a **home safety evaluation**. This professional assessment of your loved one's personal living space (whether it's in their own home or if they're living with you) can help minimize potential hazards in their environment. It is conducted by an occupational or physical therapist who will come in and assess the patient's current abilities as well as conditions in the residence.

In addition, the National Institutes of Health,[81] the Mayo Clinic,[82] and the Caregiver Support Kit produced by the National Caregiving Foundation[83] each make similar recommendations regarding potential safety issues for our elderly loved ones. These room-by-room descriptions make an excellent checklist of things every caregiver should keep a watchful eye on:

- In the kitchen:
  - ¤ Review the appliances (ease of operation, hot surface indicators, door-ajar indicators, need for childproof locks, etc.).
  - ¤ Observe chair height (either too low or too high can be a fall hazard).

80. "Home Safety Evaluation: Can I Send This Patient Home? - #22," Geriatric Fast Facts, accessed March 2022, geriatricfastfacts.com/fast-facts/home-safety-evaluation-can-i-send-patient-home

81. "Home Safety Checklist for Alzheimer's Disease," National Institute on Aging, U.S. Department of Health & Human Services, accessed March 2022, nia.nih.gov/health/home-safety-checklist-alzheimers-disease#:~:text=If%20the%20person%20with%20Alzheimer's%20is%20permitted%20in%20a%20garage,overhanging%20items%20out%20of%20reach

82. Mayo Clinic Staff, "Home Safety Tips: Preparing for Alzheimer's Caregiving," Mayo Clinic, Mayo Foundation for Medical Education and Research, accessed March 2022, mayoclinic.org/healthy-lifestyle/caregivers/in-depth/home-safety-tips/art-20046785

83. Request a Free Caregiver's Support Kit at caregivingfoundation.org/support-kit/

- ¤ Consider removing floor mats (these can be "slip" and/or "trip" hazards in *any* room of the house).
- ¤ Install a pantry lock for dangerous items (knives, scissors, etc.) and hazardous products (cleaning supplies, matches, etc.).

- In the bathroom:
  - ¤ Install a shower chair and/or grab bars.
  - ¤ Put non-skid strips or a rubber mat in the tub or shower.
  - ¤ Ask the pharmacist for child-resistant caps on all medication containers (to prevent accidental or untimely ingestion of meds).
  - ¤ Check the temperature setting on the water heater (to avoid burns from scalding water).

- In the bedroom:
  - ¤ Check the bed height (too low or too high—either extreme can cause a fall).
  - ¤ Be aware of bed placement (having the bed against a wall keeps it stationary if the patient starts to fall; the bed can help steady the patient rather than sliding away thus removing all their support).
  - ¤ Consider using a monitoring device (such as a baby monitor or security cameras).
  - ¤ Recognize threshold danger (even a minimally raised divider between rooms can be a potential trip hazard).

- In the living room:
  - ¤ Ensure that any hinged-leaf furniture (such as end tables or a dining table) is firmly locked so it won't give way if leaned on.
  - ¤ Put a decal on glass doors or windows to help the patient see the glass panes.
  - ¤ Keep furniture with sharp corners out of main walkways.
  - ¤ Trim large plants and remove any that may be poisonous if eaten.

- In the walkways, hallways, and stairwells:
  - ¤ Ensure the hall or stair paths are well-lit.
  - ¤ Keep these areas clear of any debris.
  - ¤ Make sure all stairs have a secure handrail.
  - ¤ See that electrical cords are tucked away.

- In the garage, shed, or basement:
  - ¤ If possible, lock access to these areas.
  - ¤ Install locks on cabinets where tools or sporting equipment are/is kept.

- ¤ Lock away or remove potentially dangerous items such as paint, fertilizer, gasoline, or other toxic items.
- ¤ Make sure overhanging items are out of reach.

- Miscellaneous:[84]

  - ¤ Put nightlights in the dementia patient's bedroom, bathroom, and hallways; this is particularly important if they are prone to sundowning or wandering.
  - ¤ All windows and any doors leading outside should be locked so the dementia patient doesn't accidentally wander outside (and potentially away from the house); having these exits alarmed to indicate they've been opened may also be helpful.
  - ¤ Be certain there are working smoke detectors and carbon monoxide detectors; if they are battery operated, keep track of how often the batteries need to be changed (it is recommended that you use daylight saving time as a reminder to change batteries in your detectors).
  - ¤ Maintain a safe indoor temperature (around 70 degrees is recommended); in general, older people are more vulnerable to cold, but a dementia patient may not realize how cold they are and therefore won't take proper steps to get warm.
  - ¤ Keep dishwasher and laundry detergents (including powders, liquids, and pods), fabric softeners, and bleach items locked up or stored out of sight; accidental ingestion of these poisonous items can result in death.[85]

THE LAST RESORT

"My husband and I are not anywhere near qualified to provide them with the kind of professional care they need, and Waverly was the facility that had room to take a couple. It's clean, they're safe, and they're together, and that's the best I can do!"

Excerpt from *Goodnight, Sweet: A Caregiver's Long Goodbye*
Chapter 18: "Spring"

---

84. "Home Safety Measures All Caregivers of Those with Dementia Should Know," Dementia Care Central, Developed with funding from the National Institute on Aging (Grant #R43AG026227), last updated August 14, 2020, dementiacarecentral.com/caregiverinfo/handsoncare/safety/

85. Ben Popken, "Laundry Pods Can Be Fatal for Adults With Dementia," NBC News, NBC Universal, June 16, 2017, nbcnews.com/business/consumer/laundry-pods-can-be-fatal-adults-dementia-n773366

The thought of having to place a loved one in a long-term care community such as assisted living or a nursing home can be a painful, guilt-provoking experience. Some caregivers are going to have the financial means to examine multiple options, but some caregivers won't have any other choice.

In the case of my grandparents, I had examined every possibility I could think of to avoid the nursing home, even going so far as to secure a small apartment in an independent living community. The reality, however, was that they were well past being able to live there safely; their perpetual efforts to try to get out and "go home" (although they never seemed quite sure where "home" was) kept me in a frantic state, constantly concerned they might wander off and be hurt—or worse. Grandma's Alzheimer's was well advanced, and truth be told Grandpa's unspecified dementia wasn't that much better.

I learned firsthand that many factors influenced the decision of how my grandparents would ultimately be cared for. There were certain things that overruled my desire to keep them in my home, like the level of medical care they required as well as my lack of availability—as a newly married couple at the time, neither Chris nor I could afford to quit work.

For your consideration, I've made a few notes regarding some of the common issues faced by dementia caregivers; the reality is that these situations can (and frequently do) overlap. Caregivers *are not failures* if these or other issues necessitate placing a loved one in long-term care; sometimes it's the most practical—and safest—option available.

The Wanderer

Sometimes a caregiver may be unaware of just how advanced their loved one's dementia has become, so they may think it's still safe to leave their loved one home alone for brief periods. When the dementia patient has no mobility issues, they can be out the door and gone in a matter of seconds. According to the Alzheimer's Association, **wandering** occurs with six out of ten dementia patients.[86] Several states have a Code Silver (sometimes called a Silver Alert) in place which can notify the general public to keep an eye out for a missing older adult.[87] Even with such safety measures in place, it raises concern to think of the variety of issues that could result from an elderly person wandering aimlessly.

86. "Wandering," Alzheimer's Association, accessed March 2022, alz.org/help-support/caregiving/stages-behaviors/wandering

87. Angela Stringfellow, "What Is a Code Silver? How It Works, State Information, and More," SeniorLink Blog, April 25, 2018, seniorlink.com/blog/silver-alerts#:~:text=Definition%20of%20a%20Code%20Silver,persons%20who%20have%20cognitive%20disorders

In essence, this is what happened to my grandparents, except they got in their car (rather than walking) and drove more than two hours from home where they were found four days later in their banged-up car on the side of the road. This was only one of several reasons I knew the nursing home presented a *much* safer option for them.

Medical Necessity

When my grandma was diagnosed with Alzheimer's, she was simultaneously found to be diabetic and to have a weak heart. In addition, I was told she had a poor swallow reflex which put her at a very high risk of choking every time she ate. And while she still had the ability to walk, it was very noticeable to me that she was progressively less steady on her feet, and the way she would reel when she stood up kept me on edge that she might fall, and I wouldn't be there in time to catch her.

I am not a medical professional, so knowing those issues were present, each one serious in its own right, I was very uncomfortable with the idea of trying to take care of her myself.

Anxiety

People with dementia often experience feelings of anxiety which, in turn, affects their behavior. As a general term, **anxiety** is defined as distress or uneasiness of mind caused by fear; it's something everyone experiences from time to time, but according to Harvard Medical School, anxiety symptoms are *extremely* common in dementia patients.[88]

Unaddressed anxiety can lead to agitation and aggression. Both of my grandparents experienced anxiety which caused them to behave in ways that were highly uncharacteristic of their pre-dementia personalities. Eventually they were both placed on medication (which did help), but in the back of my mind I remembered a story Grandma had told me about her own grandmother who had "outlived her mind," as Grandma put it. Her father walked in just in time to stop his mother-in-law from crashing a chair over his wife's head! I had seen enough aggression in my grandparents to realize there was no way for me to provide the care and assurance they would have needed if I had tried to keep them in my own home.

---

88. Stephanie Collier, MD, MPH, "What Works Best for Treating Depression and Anxiety in Dementia?" Harvard Health Publishing, Harvard Medical School, The President and Fellows of Harvard College, March 18, 2020, health.harvard.edu/blog/what-works-best-for-treating-depression-and-anxiety-in-dementia-2020031819071

The Caregiver's Own Health

A detailed study[89] of the mortality risk experienced by those providing prolonged care for a spouse was reported by *The Journal of the American Medical Association* (JAMA) in 1999. Participants included 392 caregivers and 427 non-caregivers aged 66–96 who were living with their spouses. In short, the study found that there was a 63 percent higher chance of caregiver death occurring due to the stress of the job than was found in their participant peers who were not caregivers. In addition, the CDC reports that more than half (53 percent) of caregivers say that because their health has declined, they feel their ability to provide care to their loved one is compromised.[90] Being the sole or main caregiver over a prolonged period of time can seriously affect both physical and mental health, so caregivers need to be aware of their limits, honestly acknowledging what they can realistically do. A long-term care community such as assisted living or a nursing home may be the better alternative for everyone involved.

When the Relationship Has Been Strained

I knew of a woman who opened her home to her aged mother when it was determined "mother" could no longer live by herself. For the next six months both the woman and her husband were utterly miserable because "mother" was so hateful to them. There were almost daily altercations that were so intense the woman literally looked for reasons not to be in her own home. Because this woman wouldn't allow her mother to completely run the house, "mother" went and complained to another relative about how unhappy *she* was. After weeks of secret planning and clandestine meetings, "mother" announced to her daughter she had found somewhere else to live; the daughter and her husband were ecstatic over the prospect of "mother" leaving because they knew it meant they would get their peaceful home back. Meanwhile, after a second failed living arrangement, "mother" wound up in a nursing home, and it was a far better situation for everyone involved. When she got ugly, it was with the nursing home staff rather than her family members who loved her but were completely unable to work with her.

89. R. Schulz & S.R. Beach, "Caregiving As a Risk Factor For Mortality: The Caregiver Health Effects Study," PubMed.gov JAMA, NIH National Library of Medicine, National Center for Biotechnology Information, December 15, 1999, pubmed.ncbi.nlm.nih.gov/10605972/

90. "Alzheimer's Disease and Healthy Aging: Caregiving; A Public Health Priority," Centers for Disease Control and Prevention, U.S. Department of Health & Human Services, accessed March 2022, cdc.gov/aging/caregiving/index.htm

The nature of the relationship between the caregiver and the one being cared for is a major consideration when looking at various care options. If there has been a contentious relationship between the parent and the adult son or daughter who's looking to take care of them, the most loving thing to do may actually be to consider assisted living or a nursing home. Ideally you want an environment where the caregiver and the one receiving care are both able to thrive. It won't be good for anyone's health to live in an atmosphere of anger and hostility.

QUESTIONS FOR CONSIDERATION

1. Do you have concerns about how steady your loved one is when they are standing or walking around?

2. If your loved one with dementia is driving and is involved in an accident that is determined to be their fault, what liability might you face as their caregiver?

3. Are you aware of the safety features and/or danger factors that are present in your loved one's living situation?

CHAPTER 6

CAREGIVER SELF-CARE: AVOIDING BURNOUT

I n this chapter we will,
- Determine why self-care is so important
- Discuss how caregiver self-care will benefit the care recipient
- Examine what healthy self-care looks like
- Recognize and manage "anticipatory grief"

One of the most common things people talk about in the twenty-first century is what amazing strides have been made in the medical field. There is an abundance of information regarding what foods to eat and which vitamins to take, what exercises to do, and how much sleep everyone should be getting in order to remain healthy and age well.

But something seems to happen to an individual when the word *caregiver* gets added to the list of roles they're already filling. It seems like all the health facts they ever heard fly right out the window when they are up to their necks in double duty—managing not only their own lives but also the finances, medical appointments, mood swings, and medications of a loved one who needs care.

It's important for caregivers to take the necessary steps to avoid burnout because once it starts, it wreaks havoc in all directions. The results of failing to practice good self-care are universally ugly, and they include (but aren't limited to) chronic stress, both physical and mental health issues, and potentially the growth of resentment toward the care recipient.

HEALTHY "ESCAPE": A HALLMARK OF SELF-CARE

Our trip to Florida was wonderfully restful. Having several days without the immediate weight of concern about Grandma and Grandpa made me realize just how weary I had grown toward everything associated with "caregiving."

Excerpt from *Goodnight, Sweet: A Caregiver's Long Goodbye*
Chapter 19: "Contact"

From day one, I had been forced to concede how bad things really were with my grandparents—*both* being diagnosed with dementia on the same day. And several weeks into my new caregiver role, I still had no comprehensive plan as to what was ultimately going to happen—even though I was very anxious to get one established. Realistically I wondered what level of care their medical conditions would ultimately demand—*and* what quality of care their savings alone could provide for them.

I slid around a frenzied learning curve as I sought to understand things like Medicare, Medicaid, and the sweeping authority granted to me by their durable power of attorney documents. I felt the pressure to make sure my grandparents were housed safely even as I was frantically trying to get all of their past-due bills caught up. I had to quickly gather a great deal of information so that two individual Medicaid applications could be completed: one for Edward and one for Clara. The hours of my day were so tied up in Meade business that I couldn't even watch a half-hour sit-com without my phone ringing; and when I answered, it was either a medical professional *making* a report or it was a relative *wanting* a report.

And just to further exacerbate my frustration, our living room had become an obstacle course with pieces of my grandparents' furniture stacked up next to our own, and scattered around the apartment were a multitude of boxes which contained a maddeningly disorganized hodge-podge of Meade paperwork. Basically, if I was awake, I was either tending to Grandma and Grandpa themselves or I was caught up in handling some part of their business. And on top of everything else, I was drifting aimlessly between a variety of emotions—sadness, depression, grief, anger, confusion, hopelessness. I felt spent right down to my core.

Even some of the medical professionals who were working with my grandparents had actually started encouraging me to take a break—an activity which began to make more sense in light of God's Word. Mark 16:31 says, "[Jesus] said to His apostles, 'Come away with me by yourselves to a quiet place and get some rest.'" As I mulled over this verse, I began to realize His instruction didn't apply exclusively to the apostles; if He cared so much about those guys that He persuaded them to get away and rest, then it's reasonable to believe He still has that same concern for us today, especially when we remember Malachi 3:6 where God says, "I the Lord do not change." Because I know He doesn't change, I believe He wants the same thing for His people today that He wanted for His apostles two thousand years ago: proper rest.

So, after months of non-stop caregiving tasks, Chris and I decided to put on the brakes. We booked a five-day trip to the beach for our first wedding anniversary, and it was there that I learned just how valuable having time away could be. Our deliberate "escape" to the shore was both restorative and energizing—a veritable "reset" button for my entire being. As I stood at the water's edge and felt the sand between my toes, I sensed my muscles beginning to relax. My heightened state of alert began to ease off, and my cloudy, confused thoughts regained a level of clarity.

But even in that relaxed environment, shades of guilt attempted to worm their way in, making me wonder if I wasn't being very selfish by lounging under a beach umbrella while my grandparents were trapped in a dementia fog, adjusting to their new life in the nursing home.

The short answer was no, I *wasn't* being selfish. If I had kept going at the pace I had originally set, it would have only been a matter of time before I would have become so worn down that I wouldn't have been able to take care of my *own* business, let alone theirs.

It's important to realize that caregiver weariness can result from not only doing things *for* a loved one but also from having to deal *with* a loved one. Consider the dementia patient's constant repetition, aimless wandering, early-evening agitation (sundowning), or outright aggression—any of these going on long enough can push a caregiver to their extreme limits.

Each care scenario is unique—and each is undeniably exhausting. Consider that some caregivers are on duty in their house 24/7; others work an eight- to ten-hour day in the business world, then go home to their *other* full-time job: that of caregiver. Still others have to schedule visits with their loved ones who live in long-term care communities such as assisted living or nursing homes.

The 24/7 caregiver can slip into an unimaginably dark depression because their "scenery" never changes. The full-time caregiver who is also a full-time employee runs the risk of total collapse by trying to keep up with the multiple responsibilities they continually shoulder. Equally difficult is the oversight of a loved one's care in assisted living or a nursing home; the caregiver's frequent visits, the facility's recurring calls—which range from incident reports to scheduling the recommended family care plan meetings—can leave the caregiver feeling completely drained.

Why is self-care so important? Because you can only keep all the plates spinning together for a short period of time; eventually something will have to give. By taking the necessary respite periods, *you* can choose which plate to briefly stop spinning rather than risk having all the plates go crashing to the ground at once.

THE WIN-WIN OF SELF-CARE

A debate ensued as to which Memphis hospital would be the best place for us to [take Grandma and Grandpa]. Presbyterian Hospital was the one [I was] the most familiar with; however, I had often heard Grandma remark that she liked the Winchester Hospital....My mother cautiously advised that Presbyterian might be better....

"We know how to get around Presbyterian. And besides... [Grandma] won't really know...."

"I just want to do for her...the way she'd want things done," [I said].

[Mom responded,] "...because she won't know the difference, it would be better to go to a place where you're familiar with the lay of the land. You're under enough pressure as it is. Don't add to that by going to a hospital you're unfamiliar with."

Excerpt from *Goodnight, Sweet: A Caregiver's Long Goodbye*
Chapter 7: "Going Home"

The quote above recounts a time we were trying to figure out how best to get my grandparents admitted to a hospital in order to meet certain Medicaid eligibility requirements. The situation was tense, and I was very anxious to "do the right thing" for my grandparents. For years I had often heard Grandma express her preference for the Winchester Hospital over Presbyterian; based on *that fact alone,* I was prepared to take them to a medical complex I knew practically nothing about. My mother was wisely suggesting I re-think my position.

I had no reason to think my grandparents would receive better care at one hospital over the other, so ultimately what difference did it make where we went? The difference would be for me, not for them; it would certainly lower *my* stress to go to a place where I was familiar with the logistics. And if my stress was lower, that had the potential to affect everything—not only how I connected with the medical professionals treating my grandparents but also how I related to Grandma and Grandpa themselves.

It's worth noting that while the durable power of attorney documents provide *authority* to make medical and financial decisions for a loved one, they make no specification about the process used by the caregiver to arrive at those decisions. That ambiguity can easily create a situation where an exhausted, overworked caregiver does something in haste without considering or realizing the possible ramifications of their choice. Depending on what the issue is, the outcome can be devastating for the care recipient. Just imagine a caregiver's decision inadvertently leading to any of the following:

- The care recipient being subjected to a medical procedure which will be physically hard on them, and may ultimately add nothing to their quality of life

- Desperately needed Medicaid being denied due to the caregiver's errors during the application process
- A weary caregiver being unintentionally short with their loved one's medical providers may find the providers' dislike of them being transferred onto the one needing care

Taking care of yourself is perhaps the greatest thing you can do in your role as a caregiver. Every task you undertake for your loved one will either be hindered or helped by *your* state of mind; both the good and the bad will ripple out from you in all directions, affecting everything in your wake. If you are mentally and physically worn-down, perpetually exhausted by the constant pull on your time and resources, the care you provide will be negatively affected. However, a caregiver who has taken steps to ensure they have healthy time away from the tasks of caregiving, along with consistently good, sound sleep and proper nutrition will be far more effective at the job. In that scenario, *everyone* wins.

READY? SET? SELF-CARE!

"I've had enough," I said evenly. "As of right now, I'm officially off duty."

**Excerpt from *Goodnight, Sweet: A Caregiver's Long Goodbye*
Chapter 18: "Spring"**

How important is it for all of us to learn to set healthy boundaries in our lives? Well, let's see: how important is good nutrition, fresh water, clean air? The answer is: healthy boundaries are a *necessity*. They bring order, and if they're not in place, life can be riddled with harmful, guilt-driven chaos.

For the caregiver, setting healthy boundaries is the very foundation of self-care. It means the caregiver is making a conscious choice to not let the burdens of the role consume every aspect of their life. It also demonstrates they will not be made to feel guilty for taking time off to manage their own affairs or even to just get away for a change of scenery once in a while.

There can be no doubt that the effects of providing care for a loved one are crushing. I didn't get very far into my own caregiving journey before I began to experience the toll—physically, mentally, and spiritually—and it was at that point I started to ponder the question, *How would it glorify God for me to let myself get all run down and worn out and possibly even fail at the task I'd been given?* Clearly there were *no* benefits to all work and no rest, so I began to search for ways to engage in proper self-care because, ultimately, I knew my grandparents needed me to be strong for their entire journey.

MAKE YOUR SLEEP A PRIORITY

If you've ever wondered whether missing a little sleep is really that big a deal, just ask the parents of a newborn. The first few weeks immediately following a baby's birth can be brutal in terms of sleep deprivation—and the new parents feel it during every second of any given twenty-four-hour period!

It's not all that different for you as a caregiver. Consider that you run, run, run all day, juggling your caregiving tasks along with your own personal activities. Before you know it, the day is nearly over, but you keep going well into the night, trying to accomplish all the things that there was no time for during the day (like cleaning your house or tending to your own finances). When you finally do get to lay down, you may find yourself too keyed up to drift off to sleep, particularly if your loved one suffers with sundowning episodes during the overnight hours. You might manage to doze off just in time for your alarm to signal the unwelcomed sound of a new day starting—and you're certain it will look just like the day before. This is an exhausting schedule and frankly one that's impossible to maintain.

There are multiple studies that clearly show how sleep-deprived people, when tested in a driving simulator, perform as badly as (or even worse than) people who are intoxicated.[91] The Cleveland Clinic states that not getting the proper amount of sleep each night can actually undermine the known health benefits of eating well and engaging in regular exercise.[92] They further state that a lack of good, sound sleep has both short- and long-term effects which initially manifest in a lack of alertness and excessive daytime sleepiness; left unchecked, sleep deprivation can lead to a variety of life-threatening conditions such as high blood pressure, heart failure, or stroke. On the other hand, healthy sleep functions as a gatekeeper which protects against a myriad of issues, including obesity, depression, and a weakened immune system.

So how much is "the proper amount" of sleep? According to the National Sleep Foundation, adults between the ages of 18 and 64 should generally try to get between seven and nine hours of sleep per night; adults over age 65 may require slightly less, but it is still recommended to strive for at least seven to eight hours of sound sleep.[93]

91. Sleep Physician at American Sleep Association Reviewers and Writers, Board-certified sleep M.D. physicians, scientists, editors and writers for ASA, "What Is Sleep and Why Is It Important?" American Sleep Association, accessed March 2022, sleepassociation. org/about-sleep/what-is-sleep/

92. "Here's What Happens When You Don't Get Enough Sleep (And How Much You Really Need a Night)," Health Essentials, Cleveland Clinic, June 16, 2020, health.cleve-landclinic.org/happens-body-dont-get-enough-sleep/#:~:text=Some%20of%20the%20 most%20serious,can%20even%20affect%20your%20appearance

93. "How Much Sleep Do You Really Need?" National Sleep Foundation, October 1, 2020, thensf.org/how-many-hours-of-sleep-do-you-really-need/

TAKE TIME OFF

One primary recommendation regarding self-care is to deliberately plan some time off from the tasks of caregiving. It's ironic that when a person is searching for a new job, one specific thing they look for in the benefits package is how much time they can take off from work and still get paid. Caregivers need to adapt a similar mindset, recognizing from the start how important it is to *intentionally* schedule time away. It may be as simple as running out for a cup of coffee while the home health nurse is working with your loved one; or maybe you can have a volunteer from your church stay with the patient for a couple of hours while you meet a friend for lunch.

People who enjoy travel need to look ahead on the calendar, clearing time over a weekend (or even in the middle of the week) *on purpose!* Actively recruit other family members to step in and help while you're gone, or check with a home health agency to see the cost involved in having staff nurses or aides stay around the clock for a couple of days.

Another idea is to plan a day trip with a friend. See what's within driving distance from your home (no more than one to two hours away), and pick a day to visit. Enjoy some great conversation and a fun lunch, and be sure to take several pictures that you can appreciate once you're home again. Go somewhere you've never been, learn something new, and snack on something from your childhood that brings a smile to your face. If it rains, don't be afraid to get wet, and if it's hot, treat yourself to an ice-cream-parlor-style milkshake; or, if it's cold, plan a stop for a warm muffin and a steaming mug of your favorite coffee or cocoa. And LAUGH at silly things with your friend! Endeavor to make the day special; your brain and your body will both thank you for the distraction.

Now, some people may argue that even if you can manage to get away, you ultimately have to come back, so what good does it really do? According to a May 2021 article published online by Forbes,[94] just taking some vacation time could actually save your life.

The article cites a recent global study conducted by the World Health Organization (WHO) which found that 745,000 people who died from heart disease and stroke in 2016 had direct links between their health conditions and their long working hours. While it's true the study focused on employees in the workforce, we need to realize that the job of a caregiver can be as labor-intensive as any work that's done for a paycheck—perhaps

94. Caroline Castrillion, "Why Taking Vacation Time Could Save Your Life," Forbes, May 23, 2021, forbes.com/sites/carolinecastrillon/2021/05/23/why-taking-vaca-tion-time-could-save-your-life/?sh=44dd020324de

even more so because the caregiver's job doesn't necessarily end after forty to fifty hours per week. The Forbes article states that "taking vacation time is essential to employee survival. That's because time off from work is integral to well-being, sustained productivity and high performance." And that's only *one* good reason to take some time off. For another, consider this: what will happen to your care recipient if something were to happen to *you*? If you are your loved one's primary caregiver and you collapse from exhaustion, who will be able to step in to fill your shoes with them for the long haul?

Make Time for Things You Enjoy

Most everyone agrees that, in general, people are over-stressed. For you as a caregiver, the normal stress levels are doubled; there are the stressors in your own personal life, and there is the continual stress you feel as a caregiver. All throughout the long, busy day, your thoughts may frequently search for ways to reduce that harmful, ever-present stress, but the tendency is to examine the same material over and over, hoping to find some new information we haven't already heard:

- Eating right—yes, we know to do that.
- Exercising—yep, we know to do that too.
- Reading—yep—wait, *what*?

That's right: reading! Studies show that it only takes six minutes of reading to lower your stress levels; as a matter of fact, research has found there is a 68 percent reduction in stress after engaging in reading fiction.[95] Empathy is cultivated when the reader's mind becomes involved in the story of the characters, so even if you don't particularly enjoy the act of reading, you might invest in some audio books. Personally I enjoy a good "whodunit," so I always recommend selecting a mystery, a real brain-teaser intermingled with well-developed characters. Download it to your phone and play it while you drive or work around the house. Don't knock it; these diversions can provide a fun, much-needed means of escape for a weary caregiver.

Maybe you love working crossword puzzles or even putting together a jigsaw puzzle; it could be knitting, gardening, or baking—whatever it may be, allow yourself time to engage in the activity that you enjoy. When you are weighed down by the responsibilities and grief of caregiving, it may seem frivolous to get involved in a "fun" activity, but allowing yourself to do that very thing can be one of the best stress relievers you'll ever have.[96]

95. "Reading Fiction for Stress Relief," De-Stress Monday, Grace Communications Foundation, March 31, 2020, mondaycampaigns.org/destress-monday/reading-fiction-stress-relief

96. Elizabeth Scott, PhD, Fact checked by Adah Chung, "Why Having Fun Provides Some of the Best Stress Relief," VeryWellMind, Dotdash Publishing, Updated June 27, 2020, verywellmind.com/the-best-stress-relief-3144573

"What Do You Feel Like You're Waiting For?"

I stared blankly for a few seconds, and then I looked straight into [Vivian's] eyes.

"We're going to die. Not today, maybe, but it's where we're headed...."

Vivian just waited silently until my gaze met hers.

"...You're experiencing a great loss that's coming in stages," [she said], "and it's left you devastated...you're experiencing [your grandparents] being 'gone' in the sense that they're not mentally who you've always known them to be. Someday they will be gone physically too, but that day's not today. Embrace them where they are....Touch them, love them, enjoy them, remember who they were. Don't put them in that casket before it's time."

Excerpt from *Goodnight, Sweet: A Caregiver's Long Goodbye*
Chapter 14: "Vivian"

These very wise words were spoken to me by my counselor, Vivian Holmes, back in 1997. She recognized what was happening to me; the longer I served as caregiver to my grandparents the more grieved I became over the changes wrought by their dementia. This, in turn, steered me down a path of distress over what those changes would eventually lead to: their deaths. So, very gently, she took my proverbial hand and led me out of the dark by offering me something substantial to hold on to: *the truth*.

The truth was that Jesus had created both of my grandparents ("For you created my inmost being; you knit me together in my mother's womb," Psalm 139:13 NIV); equally true was the fact that Jesus had numbered their days ("...all the days ordained for me were written in your book before one of them came to be," Psalm 139:16). The truth was that my grandparents *did* have dementia, and they were both going to *die* with dementia; but Vivian wanted me to know that their deaths were not imminent at that exact moment. *The real truth* was that I didn't need to be so focused on their deaths that I wound up missing the very life they were *still living*.

Dementia is a particularly vicious opponent, quite savvy at inducing a caregiver's **anticipatory grief**, which is defined as "the normal mourning that occurs when a patient or family is *expecting* a death."[97] And don't be fooled; it can be every bit as intense as the grief that follows the physical death of a loved one. While anticipatory grief can be brought on by any number of terminal diseases, dementia is uniquely cruel because it works so slowly,

---

97. Medical Editor Charles Patrick Davis, MD, PhD, "Medical Definition of Anticipatory Grief," MedicineNet, MedicineNet Inc., reviewed on March 29, 2021, medicinenet.com/anticipatory_grief/definition.htm

almost imperceptibly at first, thereby forcing the caregiver to deal with the loss in stages. As time creeps by, you suddenly realize your loved one may be physically sitting right in front of you, drawing breath, blinking, even eating a few bites of food here and there, but their vacant facial expression and the eventual lack of response to your presence all come together to reveal that their mind has been stolen away little by little, until their body's involuntary activities are all that remain to indicate they are still "alive."

Anticipatory grief is harsh because the "anticipation" part will eventually culminate in literal death—you will ultimately face the *actual passing* of your loved one, which will then force you to feel the pain of the permanent loss. But the brutality of the anticipation phase should not be underestimated. I remember having such a hard time watching my grandmother spiral down— and yet she somehow managed to keep hanging on from one day to the next. I was in full-blown grief confusion as I grappled between wanting to let her go and simultaneously wanting to hold on to her.

> *I smiled slightly, and all at once I had peace to lean over and put my cheek against hers. "It's ok, Grandma," I said directly in her ear with a voice that was barely audible. "It's ok for you to go be with Jesus...."*
>
> *But I knew in my heart that, selfishly, I still wasn't quite ready to let her go.*

Excerpt from *Goodnight, Sweet: A Caregiver's Long Goodbye*
Chapter 23: "Hello, Sweet"

Much like its conventional counterpart, anticipatory grief occurs in stages. Generally, people will experience **shock** about the upcoming loss; this is followed by **denying the reality** of the loss. Eventually **acceptance** will come,[98] but even then it's not uncommon for people to bounce back and forth between the stages. You may find that one day you're inundated with thoughts of what's coming, and other days you might be fine, not giving it any consideration at all. There may be feelings of concern for the person who is dying, and you may find you rehearse the impending death in your mind, wondering what it will feel like and what will happen at the immediate time of death. You may also find that you are trying to imagine the future, thinking about what the holidays or other special occasions will be like without your loved one.[99]

---

98. Merritt Whitley, "Anticipatory Grief: Learning the Signs and How to Cope," A Place for Mom, A Place for Mom, Inc., May 15, 2020, aplaceformom.com/caregiver-resources/articles/anticipatory-grief

99. Marissa Conrad, Medically reviewed by Judy Ho, PhD, A.B.P.P., A.B.P.D.N., "What Is Anticipatory Grief and How Does It Work?" Forbes Media, LLC, updated June 17, 2021, forbes.com/health/mind/what-is-anticipatory-grief/

One of the greatest things caregivers can do to cope with the anticipation of loss is to find a healthy way to express the pain and grief that's actually being felt. These feelings are legitimate and do not make the caregiver weak! As I have done throughout this book, I strongly urge seeing a counselor or therapist—someone who will let you sit down and process everything at your own speed. Support groups can also be very helpful as they can reduce the feelings of isolation experienced by so many caregivers. Employ the tactics discussed in the "Ready, Set, Self-Care" section: make sure you get good, sound sleep, deliberately schedule time off, and engage in doing things you enjoy.

When I found myself grieving more and more for Grandma, there were periods of time in which I found myself speechless, unable to adequately express the cry of my heart for her. What brought me comfort was Romans 8:26 (AMP):

In the same way the Spirit [comes to us and] helps us in our weakness. We do not know what prayer to offer or how to offer it as we should, but the Spirit Himself [knows our need and at the right time] intercedes on our behalf with sighs and groanings too deep for words.

I began to understand that God doesn't anoint us and give us His Spirit for the "easy" times in our lives. Instead, He equips us to withstand great difficulties; it is during these hard experiences that we find He gives us not only His grace, but He gives us Himself as well:

God is our refuge and strength, an ever-present help in trouble. Therefore, we will not fear, though the earth give way and the mountains fall into the heart of the sea, though its waters roar and foam and the mountains quake with their surging. (Psalm 46:1-3 NIV)

QUESTIONS FOR CONSIDERATION

1. If you suddenly become overwhelmed by the enormity of your caregiving duties, who would be your "backup caregiver" to take over your responsibilities?

2. What are some things *you can do right now* to prevent caregiver burn-out?

3. How can you prepare yourself to transition from anticipatory grief to the conventional grief that follows a death?

GLOSSARY OF TERMS

advance directive – a legal document in which the signer gives directions or designates another person to make decisions regarding the signer's health care if the signer becomes incapable of making such decisions.[1]

Alzheimer's Disease – the most common type of dementia; it is a specific progressive disease of the brain that slowly causes impairment in memory and cognitive function. It is *not* a regular part of aging.[2]

anticipatory grief – grief that occurs *before* death; it is common among people facing the eventual death of a loved one or their own death. Most people expect to feel grief *after* a death, but fewer are familiar with grief that shows up before a life ends.[3]

beneficiary – (in law) the person designated to receive the income of an estate that is subject to a trust; or, the person named (as in an insurance policy) to receive proceeds or benefits.[4]

clinical driving assessment – one category of a professional driving assessment in which a trained professional evaluates driving abilities; it includes a review of medical history and cognitive assessment, functional/on-road assessment, and recommendations regarding treatment and intervention.[5]

community spouse – (also called the *well spouse* or *non-applicant spouse*) is the spouse of an individual who is receiving Medicaid-funded long-term care in an institutional setting such as a nursing home.[6]

Community Spouse Resource Allowance (CSRA) – If only one spouse requires long-term care in a facility such as a nursing home, Medicaid allows protection for the couple's assets, financial resources, and income which provides for the community spouse so that he or she will not be living in poverty.[7]

CT (computerized tomography) **scan** – a scan which combines a series of X-ray images taken from different angles around your body and uses computer processing to create cross-sectional images (slices) of the bones, blood vessels, and soft tissues inside your body. CT scan images provide more detailed information than plain X-rays do.[8]

dementia – an "umbrella" term for several different diseases affecting memory, other cognitive abilities, and behavior; the effects of these diseases are severe enough to interfere with a person's ability to maintain their activities of daily living. It is *not* a normal part of aging.[9]

dementia with Lewy bodies (also known as Lewy body dementia or LBD) – a disease associated with abnormal deposits of a protein called alpha-synuclein in the brain. These deposits, called Lewy bodies, affect chemicals in the brain whose changes, in turn, can lead to problems with thinking, movement, behavior, and mood.[10]

do not resuscitate (DNR) **order** – a medical order which instructs health care providers not to do cardiopulmonary resuscitation (CPR) if a patient's breathing stops or if the patient's heart stops beating.[11]

driving skills evaluation – one category of a professional driving assessment in which a trained professional evaluates driving abilities; it's an in-car evaluation conducted by state-licensed and trained driving instructors. It helps drivers identify any weaknesses in driving skills and determine if supplemental training can further reduce driving risk.[12]

durable medical equipment (DME) – equipment and supplies ordered by a health care provider for everyday or extended use.[13]

durable power of attorney (POA) – a legal document designating an agent to act on behalf of the person signing the document (the "principal"), that remains in effect if the principal becomes incapacitated.[14]

executor – (in law) a person named in a deceased person's will to carry out the provisions of that will.[15]

executrix – (in law) a woman named in a deceased person's will to carry out the provisions of that will.[16]

Falls Risk Assessment – used by medical providers to find out if a patient has a low, moderate, or high risk of falling.[17]

federal tax law – the legal "rules" for how much the state, local, and federal governments can charge you for taxes each year; it also covers the procedures, policies, and penalties for everything to do with tax issues.[18]

financial means – one criterion of Medicaid eligibility; it requires a Medicaid applicant to have assets consistent with state-defined thresholds.[19]

financial power of attorney – a legal document that lets you appoint someone to manage your finances and property for you.[20]

frontotemporal dementia (FTD) – a group of disorders that occur when nerve cells in the frontal and temporal lobes of the brain are lost, causing the lobes to shrink; FTD can affect behavior, personality, language, and movement.[21]

functionality – one criterion of Medicaid eligibility; it refers to a Medicaid applicant meeting state-defined functional eligibility criteria, which are based on the applicant's physical and cognitive abilities.[22]

guardianship/conservatorship – Guardianship refers to the legal role given to an individual to manage the personal activities or resources of another person who cannot properly do so on their own. It can refer to either the care of a child or to the care of an adult when a court determines that the adult has a disability preventing them from exercising judgment (in reference to adult care, this is also called conservatorship).[23]

health care – as two separate words, it's defined as the efforts made by trained and licensed professionals to maintain or restore well-being.[24]

healthcare – as one word, it's defined as the business, institution, or activity offering medical services.[25]

Health Insurance Portability and Accountability Act of 1996 (HIPAA) – a federal law that required the creation of national standards to protect sensitive patient health information from being disclosed without the patient's consent or knowledge.[26]

home safety evaluation – an assessment of a patient's home living environment with a goal of increasing the safety of the home for the elderly person who resides there; it is conducted in the home by either a physical or an occupational therapist.[27]

incompetent – unable to manage one's affairs due to mental incapacity or sometimes physical disability; incompetence can be the basis for the appointment of a guardian or conservator to handle the incapacitated person's affairs.[28]

intestate – *Intestacy* is the state of dying without a will; if a person dies without a will, he is said to have "died intestate."[29]

last will and testament – a document written by a person (known as the testator) that details what is to happen to property owned by that person upon their death; the term *will* is also used to refer to the same document, though to be precise, a *last will and testament* refers to the most recent version of a will.[30]

living trust – an estate planning tool that bypasses probate; the trust will hold a person's assets during their lifetime and allow them to be distributed to the heirs upon the person's death; compared to a will, a living trust can often get inheritances to the beneficiaries more quickly.[31]

living will – a legal document that is used to instruct care providers in the event that you can no longer make decisions for yourself; it can shield your loved ones from having to make difficult choices about your care and reduces the chances of confusion or arguments over what's in your best interest.[32]

Medicaid – a program that provides health coverage to millions of Americans, including eligible low-income adults, children, pregnant women, elderly adults, and people with disabilities; it is jointly funded by individual states and the federal government. It does cover long-term care.[33]

Medicaid Estate Recovery Program (MERP) – a program whereby Medicaid may take its money back from the estate of a Medicaid enrollee who is 55 or older once the enrollee is deceased; it's a recovery of the money Medicaid spent on the enrollee's care.[34]

Medicaid regulations – this refers to the rules that govern Medicaid; these regulations include eligibility requirements as well as the services that are covered.[35]

medical necessity – "proof" requirements will vary by state, but in general terms, the Medicaid applicant, in order to be accepted into the program, must demonstrate a medical condition which has care needs that go beyond what an untrained person can provide, thus necessitating physician/licensed nursing staff oversight in an institutional setting (such as a nursing home).[36]

medical power of attorney (POA) – a legal document designating an agent to act on behalf of the person signing the document (the "principal"); the medical POA specifically grants the designated agent authority to step in and make *medical* decisions for the principal if they become too ill or are otherwise incapacitated and can't make those decisions on their own.[37]

Medicare – a federally funded medical insurance program for people who are 65 or older (Medicare may also cover certain people who are under 65 with disabilities).[38]

Medicare Part A – in general terms, Part A provides hospital insurance for the Medicare recipient; this can include inpatient care in hospitals or a short-term stay at a skilled nursing facility, hospice care, and home health care.[39]

Medicare Part B – in general terms, Part B provides medical insurance for the Medicare recipient; this can include services from doctors and other health care providers, outpatient care, home health care, durable medical equipment, and many preventative services like yearly "wellness" visits.[40]

Medigap – a Medicare supplemental insurance that helps fill the "gaps" in original Medicare; it's sold by private companies.[41]

memory care – a form of residential long-term care that provides intensive, specialized care for people with memory issues.[42]

minimum monthly maintenance needs allowance (MMMNA) – Medicaid's financial allowance for the spouse of a Medicaid nursing home applicant; its purpose is to ensure the non-applicant spouse will have sufficient income to live on.[43]

monthly housing allowance – Medicaid's financial allowance for the spouse of a Medicaid nursing home applicant; it makes funds available for the community spouse to cover expenses such as rent, mortgage, property taxes, and homeowners' insurance.[44]

MRI (Magnetic Resonance Imaging) – a noninvasive test doctors use to diagnose medical conditions. It uses a powerful magnetic field, radiofrequency pulses, and a computer to produce detailed pictures of internal body structures; it does not use radiation (X-rays).[45]

non-durable power of attorney - the agent's power to act ends if the principal becomes incapacitated; a non-durable POA would therefore not be useful for estate planning.[46]

Parkinson's Disease Dementia – a decline in thinking and reasoning that develops in many people living with Parkinson's at least a year after diagnosis; changes caused by Parkinson's disease begin in an area of the brain that plays a key role in movement which leads to early symptoms that include tremors and shakiness, muscle stiffness, shuffling steps, stooped posture, difficult initiating movement, and lack of facial expression.[47]

payable on death (POD) – an arrangement between a bank or credit union and their client that designates beneficiaries to receive all of the client's assets; the immediate transfer of assets is triggered by the death of the client.[48]

PET scan (Positron Emission Tomography) – in general terms, it's an imaging test that allows doctors to check for disease; it uses a special dye containing radioactive tracers which will collect in areas of higher chemical activity in the body.[49]

Probate – a court-supervised procedure of administering a will; it determines if a deceased person's will is valid and authentic, pays off their debts, and properly transfers their property to their heirs.[50]

Professional Driving Assessment – intended to serve as a "check-up" for driving skills, the professional driving assessment has two categories: driving skills evaluations and clinical driving assessments.[51]

settlor – the party that creates a trust; the settlor transfers the legal title of an asset to the trustee (the party that oversees the trust; this could be a bank or an attorney). The trustee then makes sure that the trust property is used for the beneficiary (the party that benefits from the trust).[52]

Silver Alert (also known as a *Code Silver*) – a program that sends out an alert to help find older adults who are missing, particularly those who have Alzheimer's or other forms of dementia; it can also be used for missing persons who have cognitive disorders.[53]

statutory durable power of attorney – a power of attorney document that copies the language in a state statute; the provisions of the statutory power of attorney are provided by the laws of the particular state in which it's drafted. Being "durable" means the document is unaffected by incapacitation of the principal.[54]

sundowning – restlessness, agitation, irritability, or confusion experienced by dementia patients (particularly those with Alzheimer's disease) that can begin or worsen as daylight begins to fade; it can continue into the night, making it hard for these patients to fall asleep and stay in bed.[55]

trustee – the party who holds legal title to the trust property (this is the person who has been appointed by the settlor to oversee the trust for the beneficiary).[56]

vascular cognitive impairment – a term encompassing vascular dementia as well as milder forms of pre-dementia cognitive impairment related to vascular damage that do not meet the criteria for a diagnosis of dementia.[57]

vascular dementia – a decline in thinking skills caused by conditions that block or reduce blood flow to various regions of the brain, depriving them of oxygen and nutrients.[58]

ENDNOTES

1   The Free Dictionary, Farlex, Inc., accessed April 2022, thefreedictionary.com/advance+directive

2   Daniel Yetman, medically reviewed by Shilpa Amin, M.D., CAQ, FAAFP, *Healthline*, Healthline Media, updated December 22, 2021, healthline.com/health/alzheimers-disease/difference-dementia-alzheimers

3   Lynne Eldridge, MD, medically reviewed by Adjoa Smalls-Mantey, MD, DPhil, verywellhealth, Dotdash Media, Inc., updated November 5, 2021, verywellhealth.com/understanding-anticipatory-grief-and-symptoms-2248855

4   Merriam-Webster, Inc., accessed April 2022, merriam-webster.com/dictionary/beneficiary

5   AAA Exchange, AAA, accessed April 2022, exchange.aaa.com/safety/senior-driver-safety-mobility/evaluate-your-driving-ability/

6   "How Couple's Joint Assets Impact Medicaid Eligibility," Paying for Senior Care, accessed April 2022, payingforseniorcare.com/medicaid/joint-assets-impact-eligibility#:~:text=Community%20Spouse%20%E2%80%93%20A%20community%20spouse,Services%20(HCBS)%20Medicaid%20Waiver

7   "Medicaid's Community Spouse Resource Allowance (CSRA): Calculations and Limits," American Council on Aging, accessed April 2022, medicaidplanningassistance.org/community-spouse-resource-allowance/

8   "CT Scan," Mayo Clinic, Mayo Foundation for Medical Education and Research, accessed April 2022, mayoclinic.org/tests-procedures/ct-scan/about/pac-20393675

9   "Dementia," World Health Organization, accessed April 2022, who.int/health-topics/dementia#tab=tab_1

10 "What Is Lewy Body Dementia? Causes, Symptoms, and Treatments," National Institute on Aging, U.S. Department of Health & Human Services, accessed April 2022, nia.nih.gov/health/what-lewy-body-dementia-causes-symptoms-and-treatments#:~:text=Lewy%20body%20dementia%20(LBD)%20is,movement%2C%20behavior%2C%20and%20mood

11 "Do-not-resuscitate Order," Medline Plus, National Library of Medicine, National Institutes of Health, updated April 1, 2022, medlineplus.gov/ency/patientinstructions/000473.htm

12 AAA Exchange, AAA, accessed April 2022, exchange.aaa.com/safety/senior-driver-safety-mobility/evaluate-your-driving-ability/

13 "Durable Medical Equipment (DME), HealthCare.gov, USA.gov, accessed April 2022, healthcare.gov/glossary/durable-medical-quipment-dme/

14 Content Team, "Durable Power of Attorney," Legal Dictionary, January 1, 2015, legaldictionary.net/durable-power-of-attorney/

15 Dictionary.com, accessed April 2022, dictionary.com/browse/executor

16 Dictionary.com, accessed April 2022, dictionary.com/browse/executrix

17   Medline Plus, National Library of Medicine, National Institutes of Health, updated September 13, 2021, medlineplus.gov/lab-tests/fall-risk-assessment/#:~:text=A%20fall%20 risk%20assessment%20is,reduce%20the%20chance%20of%20injury

18   Findlaw.com, Thomson Reuters, accessed April 2022, findlaw.com/tax. html#:~:text=Tax%20law%20is%20the%20legal,to%20do%20with%20tax%20issues

19   "Chapter 4: Functional Assessments for Long-Term Services and Supports," PDF, Page 3, accessed April 2022, macpac.gov/wp-content/uploads/2016/06/Functional-Assessments-for-Long-Term-Services-and-Supports.pdf

20   "What Is a Financial Power of Attorney?" FreeWill, FreeWill Co., accessed April 2022, freewill.com/learn/what-is-a-durable-financial-power-of-attorney#:~:text=A%20financial%20power%20of%20attorney%20is%20a%20legal%20document%20 that,your%20insurance%20benefits%2C%20and%20more

21   "Frontotemporal Dementia," Johns Hopkins Medicine, The Johns Hopkins University, The Johns Hopkins Hospital and Johns Hopkins Health System, accessed April 2022, hopkinsmedicine.org/health/conditions-and-diseases/dementia/frontotemporal-dementia#:~:text=Frontotemporal%20dementia%20(FTD)%2C%20 a,personality%2C%20language%2C%20and%20movement

22   "Chapter 4: Functional Assessments for Long-Term Services and Supports," PDF, Page 3, accessed April 2022, macpac.gov/wp-content/uploads/2016/06/Functional-Assessments-for-Long-Term-Services-and-Supports.pdf

23   "Guardianship," Legal Information Institute, Cornell Law School, accessed April 2022, law.cornell.edu/wex/guardianship

24   "Healthcare vs. Health Care – Which One Is It?" Grammarist, accessed April 2022, grammarist.com/spelling/healthcare/

25   "Healthcare vs. Health Care – Which One Is It?" Grammarist, accessed April 2022, grammarist.com/spelling/healthcare/

26   "Health Insurance Portability and Accountability Act of 1996 (HIPAA)," Public Health Professionals' Gateway, Public Health Law, Centers for Disease Control and Prevention, U.S. Department of Health & Human Services, accessed April 2022, cdc.gov/phlp/publications/topic/hipaa.html

27   "Home Safety Evaluation: Can I send this patient home? - #22," Geriatric Fast Facts, accessed April 2022, geriatricfastfacts.com/fast-facts/home-safety-evaluation-can-i-send-patient-home#:~:text=A%20Home%20Safety%20Evaluation%20is,patient%20 while%20in%20the%20home

28   Legal Information Institute, Cornell Law School, accessed April 2022, law.cornell.edu/ wex/incompetent

29   Legal Information Institute, Cornell Law School, accessed April 2022, law.cornell.edu/ wex/intestacy

30   Legal Information Institute, Cornell Law School, accessed April 2022, law.cornell.edu/ wex/last_will_and_testament

31   Jane Haskins, Esq., "What Does a Living Trust Do?" Legal Zoom, Legalzoom.com, Inc. updated March 17, 2022, legalzoom.com/articles/what-does-a-living-trust-do

32   LegalZoom Staff, "What Is a Living Will?" Legal Zoom, LegalZoom.com, Inc., updated March 17, 2022, legalzoom.com/articles/what-is-a-living-will

33   "Medicaid," Medicaid.gov, Centers for Medicare & Medicaid Services, accessed April 2022, medicaid.gov/medicaid/index.html

34 Elizabeth Davis, RN, Fact checked by Elaine Hinzey, RD, "How Medicaid Takes Its Money Back After You Die," verywellhealth, Dotdash Media, Inc., updated November 25, 2020, verywellhealth.com/how-the-medicaid-estate-recovery-program-works-1738836

35 "Reference Guide to Federal Medicaid Statute and Regulations," MACPAC, Medicaid and CHIP Payment and Access Commission, accessed April 2022, macpac.gov/reference-materials/reference-guide-to-federal-medicaid-statute-and-regulations/

36 "How Is Medical Necessity Determined for Medicaid Nursing Home Care?" The Hale Law Firm, accessed April 2022, thehalelawfirm.com/faqs/how-is-medical-necessity-determined-for-medicaid-nursing-home-care/

37 Belle Wong, "What Is Medical Power of Attorney?" Legal Zoom, LegalZoom.com, Inc., updated August 2, 2021, legalzoom.com/articles/what-is-medical-power-of-attorney

38 "What's Medicare?" PDF, Department of Health & Human Services, revised April 2020, medicare.gov/Pubs/pdf/11306-Medicare-Medicaid.pdf

39 "What's Medicare?" PDF, Department of Health & Human Services, revised April 2020, medicare.gov/Pubs/pdf/11306-Medicare-Medicaid.pdf

40 "What's Medicare?" PDF, Department of Health & Human Services, revised April 2020, medicare.gov/Pubs/pdf/11306-Medicare-Medicaid.pdf

41 "What's Medicare Supplement Insurance (Medigap)?" Medicare.gov, U.S. Centers for Medicare and Medicaid Services, accessed April 2022, medicare.gov/supplements-other-insurance/whats-medicare-supplement-insurance-medigap

42 Michelle Crouch, "Memory Care: Specialized Support for People with Alzheimer's or Dementia," AARP, updated December 6, 2021, aarp.org/caregiving/basics/info-2019/memory-care-alzheimers-dementia.html

43 "How Medicaid's Minimum Monthly Maintenance Needs Allowance Works & 2022 Limits," American Council on Aging, updated February 14, 2022, medicaidplanningassistance.org/mmmna-definition/#:~:text=The%20Community%20Spouse%20Monthly%20Housing,taxes%2C%20and%20homeowners'%20insurance

44 "How Medicaid's Minimum Monthly Maintenance Needs Allowance Works & 2022 Limits," American Council on Aging, updated February 14, 2022, medicaidplanningassistance.org/mmmna-definition/#:~:text=The%20Community%20Spouse%20Monthly%20Housing,taxes%2C%20and%20homeowners'%20insurancemedicaidplanningassistance.org/mmmna-definition/#:~:text=The%20Community%20Spouse%20Monthly%20Housing,taxes%2C%20and%20homeowners'%20insurance

45 "Body MRI," RadiologyInfo.org, Sponsored by American College of Radiology and Radiological Society of North America, accessed April 2022, radiologyinfo.org/en/info/bodymr

46 "Five Types of Power of Attorney Explained," Freewill, Freewill, Co., accessed April 2022, freewill.com/learn/5-types-of-power-of-attorney

47 "Parkinson's Disease Dementia," Alzheimer's Association, accessed April 2022, alz.org/alzheimers-dementia/what-is-dementia/types-of-dementia/parkinson-s-disease-dementia

48 Julia Kagan, reviewed by Roger Wohlner, fact checked by Ariel Courage, "Payable On Death (POD)," Investopedia, Dotdash Meredith Publishing Family, updated September 28, 2020, investopedia.com/terms/p/payableondeath.asp#:~:text=Payable%20on%20death%20(POD)%20is,structures%20are%20important%20to%20understand

49 Brian Krans, medically reviewed by Megan Soliman, MD, "What Is a Positron Emission Tomography (PET) Scan?" Healthline, Healthline Media, updated December 16, 2021, healthline.com/health/pet-scan

50 Catherine Hodder, Esq., reviewed by Tim Kelly, J.D., "What Is Probate?" FindLaw, Thomson Reuters, updated September 20, 2021, findlaw.com/estate/probate/what-is-probate-.html

51 AAA Exchange, AAA, accessed April 2022, exchange.aaa.com/safety/senior-driver-safety-mobility/evaluate-your-driving-ability/

52 Legal Information Institute, Cornell Law School, accessed April 2022, law.cornell.edu/wex/settlor

53 Angela Stringfellow, "What Is a Code Silver? How It Works, State Information and More," Seniorlink Blog, April 25, 2018, seniorlink.com/blog/silver-alerts#:~:text=Definition%20of%20a%20Code%20Silver,persons%20who%20have%20cognitive%20disorders

54 "Statutory Power of Attorney Law and Legal Definition," USLegal.com, airSlate Legal Forms, Inc., d/b/a USLegal, accessed April 2022, definitions.uslegal.com/s/statutory-power-of-attorney/

55 "Alzheimer's Caregiving: Tips for Coping with Sundowning," National Institute on Aging, U.S. Department of Health & Human Services, accessed April 2022, nia.nih.gov/health/tips-coping-sundowning#:~:text=They%20may%20experience%20sundowning%E2%80%94restlessness,asleep%20and%20stay%20in%20bed

56 Legal Information Institute, Cornell Law School, accessed April 2022, law.cornell.edu/wex/trustee

57 Dr. Anne M. Bonnici-Mallia, et al., "Vascular Cognitive Impairment and Vascular Dementia," Sage Journals Abstract, accessed April 2022, journals.sagepub.com/doi/10.1177/1755738018760649

58 "Vascular Dementia," Alzheimer's Association, accessed April 2022, alz.org/alzheimers-dementia/what-is-dementia/types-of-dementia/vascular-dementia

MORE FROM LEAH STANLEY

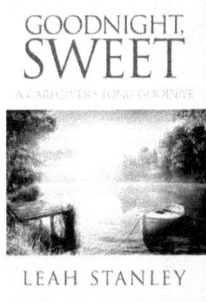

Goodnight, Sweet: A Caregiver's Long Goodbye

This book recounts Leah Stanley's unexpected and heart-wrenching journey as the primary caregiver for her aging grandparents who both developed dementia. She loved her grandparents and did her best to help them, but she was young and naïve, and her journey could rightly be described as the proverbial "trial by fire." Years later, a little older and a little wiser, she would walk a different version of this path again with her parents, but she discovered she still had a lot to learn. Through it all, God has directed her path and covered her weaknesses with His grace, and she believes that perhaps He allowed her to walk this journey so that she might be a help to others. **Access this book here.**

Caring for a Loved One with Alzheimer's or Other Dementia — **Quick Reference Guide**

This brief guide includes an abridged version of material used in the course and the unabridged eBook. This guide focuses on the essential points that you need right now, but it has many links so you can learn more on any topic of immediate interest.

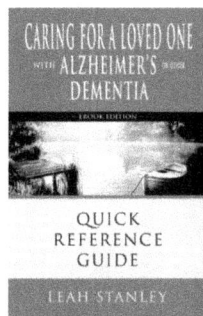

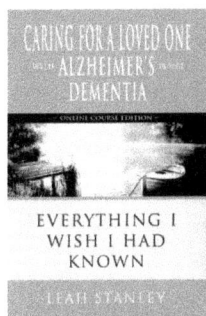

Caring for a Loved One with Alzheimer's or Other Dementia — **Online Course Editions**

The contents of this book have been incorporated into two online courses:

1. **The Professional Continuing Education (CE) Caregiver Course** is certified for social workers, nurses, and certified case managers. The course covers the day-to-day needs and available resources for primary caregivers of loved ones with Alzheimer's or other dementia. To learn more and take this course, scan the QR code or place the following link into your browser: https://bit.ly/ce-course

2. **The Individual & Healthcare Organization Caregiver Course** is designed for individuals caring for a loved one and for healthcare staffers who want to be prepared to support their organization's clients who are primary caregivers (but don't need the continuing education credit). The course can be accessed by individuals, or group registration can be arranged. To learn more and take this course, scan the QR code or place the link below into your browser: https://bit.ly/caregiver-course

www.ingramcontent.com/pod-product-compliance
Lightning Source LLC
Chambersburg PA
CBHW052104270326
41931CB00012B/2886